Clinical Cases in Dermatology

Series Editor

Robert A. Norman
Tampa, FL, USA

This series of concise practical guides is designed to facilitate the clinical decision-making process by reviewing a number of cases and defining the various diagnostic and management decisions open to clinicians.

Each title is illustrated and diverse in scope, enabling the reader to obtain relevant clinical information regarding both standard and unusual cases in a rapid, easy to digest format. Each focuses on one disease or patient group, and includes common cases to allow readers to know they are doing things right if they follow the case guidelines.

More information about this series at http://www.springer.com/series/10473

Torello Lotti • Michael Tirant • Uwe Wollina
Editors

Clinical Cases in Melanoma

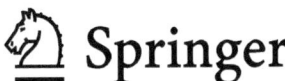

Editors
Torello Lotti
Dermatology
University of Rome Guglielmo Marconi
Roma
Roma
Italy

Michael Tirant
Dermatology
University of Rome Guglielmo Marconi
Roma
Roma
Italy

Uwe Wollina
Dermatologie und Allergologie
Städtisches Klinikum Dresden
Dresden
Sachsen
Germany

ISSN 2730-6178   ISSN 2730-6186   (electronic)
Clinical Cases in Dermatology
ISBN 978-3-030-50819-7   ISBN 978-3-030-50820-3   (eBook)
https://doi.org/10.1007/978-3-030-50820-3

This Springer imprint is published by the registered company Springer Nature Switzerland AG
The registered company address is: Gewerbestrasse 11, 6330 Cham, Switzerland

Contents

Chapter 1
Odd Looking Nail

Marija Delaš Aždajić, Mirna Šitum, Majda Vučić, and Marija Buljan

A 57-year-old Caucasian woman was examined due to a 3-year history of a pigmented, longitudinal streak involving the nail plate of her left index finger (Fig. 1.1), with no history of trauma to the digit. Clinical examination did not reveal any sign of nail destruction, while dermoscopic examination demonstrated unevenly pigmented, longitudinal lines along the entire nail plate, with pigmentation extending to the distal nail fold (Fig. 1.2).

Based on the case description and the photographs, what is your diagnosis?

1. Subungual hematoma
2. Acral lentiginous melanoma
3. Pigmented nevus
4. Onychomycosis
5. Malnutrition induced hyperpigmentation

M. D. Aždajić (✉)
Department of Dermatology and Venereology, Sestre Milosrdnice University Hospital Center, Zagreb, Croatia
e-mail: marija.delas.azdajic@kbcsm.hr

M. Šitum · M. Buljan
Department of Dermatology and Venereology, Sestre Milosrdnice University Hospital Center, Zagreb, Croatia

School of Dental Medicine, University of Zagreb, Zagreb, Croatia
e-mail: mirna.situm@kbcsm.hr; marija.buljan@kbxsm.hr

M. Vučić
School of Dental Medicine, University of Zagreb, Zagreb, Croatia

Division of Pathology and Citology "Ljudevit Jurak", Sestre Milosrdnice University Hospital Center, Zagreb, Croatia
e-mail: majda.vucic@kbcsm.hr

T. Lotti et al. (eds.), *Clinical Cases in Melanoma*,
Clinical Cases in Dermatology, https://doi.org/10.1007/978-3-030-50820-3_1

Fig. 1.1 Left index finger: initial clinical presentation

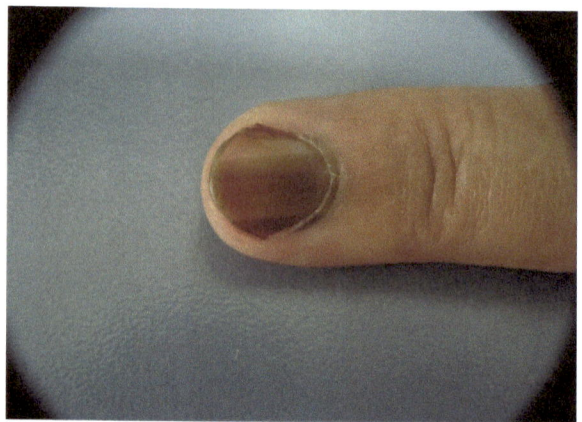

Fig. 1.2 Initial dermoscopy: unevenly pigmented, longitudinal lines along the entire nail plate, with pigmentation extending to the distal nail fold and partial nail dystrophy

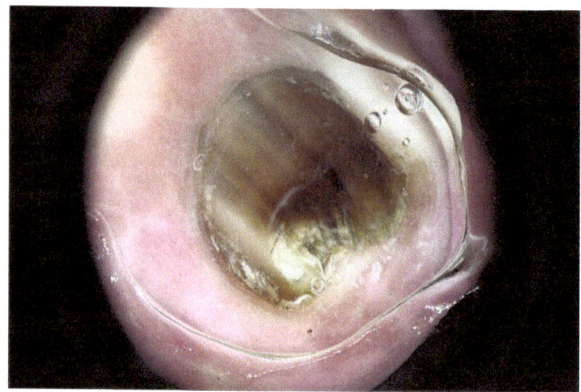

A nail matrix biopsy was performed, and histopathological analysis revealed only focal hyperpigmented epithelial basal layer without cell atypia. Due to the progression of atypical periungual pigmentation and partial nail dystrophy, a skin biopsy was repeated two more times, again, without histopathological confirmation of melanocytes.

During the following months, the discoloration and nail dystrophy progressed. Total avulsion of the nail unit with Blair-Brown skin-graft was performed and histopathological analysis at that time demonstrated atypical melanocytes, irregularly distributed without nest formation, which confirmed the diagnosis of acral lentiginous melanoma in situ (Fig. 1.3), with 5 mm clear margins. Of note, the atypical melanocytes were positive for HMB-45.

The patient has been under regular follow-up for the past 2 years, with no signs of recurrence.

Fig. 1.3 Clinical
presentation after the
surgical resection

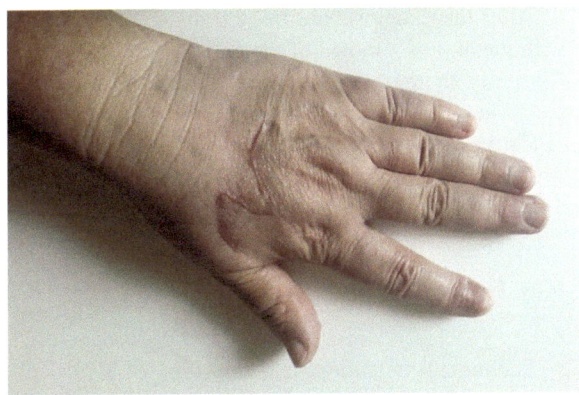

Diagnosis

Acral lentiginous melanoma.

Discussion

Acral lentiginous melanomas (ALMs) are the least common variant of melanomas, commonly found on the palms, soles and nail-beds. Subungual melanoma (SM) is a rare type of ALM that arises from the nail matrix and usually presents as melanonychia striata, with or without nail dystrophy. SM is a result of the development of malignant melanocytes along the basal layer of the epidermis, followed by development of the Hutchinson sign which is considered to be an important clue to the diagnosis [1].

This type of melanoma is commonly misdiagnosed by clinicians, indicating that early recognition and diagnosis lead to a better outcome. Additionally, histopathological picture of early stage of SM is often difficult to differentiate from benign melanocytic lesions, such as pigmented nevus [2].

If the lesion is suspicious of SM, the incisional biopsy should be performed. However, this type of biopsy might be insufficient, causing a misleading of the correct diagnosis. Longitudinal incisional biopsy of a lesion suspicious of SM should be performed after detailed dermoscopic examination, sometimes even several biopsies should be taken from multiple sites, as a single site biopsy could miss a malignant focus [3, 4].

Additionally, the pathological diagnosis of SM can be challenging, and histopathological findings may not correspond to clinical diagnosis. Therefore, clinical examination and continuous follow-up of the patient along with digital dermoscopy followed by appropriate nail matrix biopsy are crucial in reaching the correct diagnosis [5].

After the diagnosis has been confirmed, surgical resection should be performed with the aim of removal of the entire primary lesion with satisfactory free margins. Currently, there is no standardized surgical approach for treatment of SM, however, recent publications in the literature propose non-amputative, conservative treatment of SM in situ lesions, with the aim of preserving full functionality of the digit as it was performed in our patient [6, 7].

Key Points

- Subungual melanoma is a rare type of acral lentiginous melanoma that arises from the nail matrix and usually presents as longitudinal melanonychia.
- Early diagnosis and treatment play important role in the patient outcome.
- Recent publications provide evidence of safety and effectiveness of conservative surgical, non-amputative treatment for early SM.

References

1. Boriani F, O'Leary F, Tohill M, Orlando A. Acral Lentiginous Melanoma – misdiagnosis, referral delay and 5 years specific survival according to site. Eur Rev Med Pharmacol Sci. 2014;18(14):1990–6.
2. Calonje JE, Brenn T, McKee ALP. McKee's pathology of the skin: with clinical correlations. 4th ed. Philadelphia, PA: Elsevier/Saunders; 2011.
3. Chow WT, Bhat W, Magdub S, Orlando A. In situ subungual melanoma: digit salvaging clearance. J Plast Reconstr Aesthet Surg. 2013;66(2):274–6.
4. Cochran AM, Buchanan PJ, Bueno RA Jr, Neumeister MW. Subungual melanoma: a review of current treatment. Plast Reconstr Surg. 2014;134(2):259–73.
5. Levit EK, Kagen MH, Scher RK, Grossman M, Altman E. The ABC rule for clinical detection of subungual melanoma. J Am Acad Dermatol. 2000;42(2):269–74.
6. Sinno S, Wilson S, Billig J, Shapiro R, Choi M. Primary melanoma of the hand: an algorithmic approach to surgical management. J Plast Surg Hand Surg. 2015;49(6):339–45.
7. Wolff K, Goldsmith LA, Katz SI, Gilchrest BA, Paller AS, Leffell DJ. Fitzpatrick's dermatology in general medicine. 7th ed. New York, NY: McGraw Hill Medical; 2008.

Chapter 2
Serious Adverse Event Caused by Combined Target Therapy

Sanja Poduje, Jasmina Marić Brozić, Ivana Prkačin, Marija Delaš Aždajić, and Andy Goren

A 38-year old Caucasian male presented to our clinic with lymphadenopathy in left axillar region and abdominal region. Left axillar lymph node biopsy confirmed metastatic melanoma with V600E mutation in *BRAF* but no evidence of primary tumour. Patients' history revealed complete excision of nevus in the scapular region 5 years ago, and pathohistological revision confirmed dysplastic composite nevus with surrounding halo.

Positron emission tomography-computed tomography (PET-CT) identified enlarged and atypical lymph nodes located in several regions: left axilla, spleen, pancreas and para-aortic retroperitoneal region. Fine-needle aspiration in the projection of pancreas confirmed wide-spread metastatic disease. Due to overall good condition and low tumour load, immunotherapy treatment with pembrolisumab was a chosen treatment option. After the initial positive response, control PET-CT 6 months after the introduction of therapy revealed disease progression and the immunotherapy was discontinued.

A second line therapy with vemarufenib plus cobimetinib was initiated. One week after the beginning of combined target therapy, the patient developed an insignificant maculopapular rash on the trunk and extremities (Fig. 2.1). A short course

S. Poduje · I. Prkačin · M. D. Aždajić (✉)
Department of Dermatology and Venereology, Sestre Milosrdnice University Hospital Center, Zagreb, Croatia
e-mail: sanja.poduje@kbcsm.hr; ivana.prkacin@kbcsm.hr; marija.delas.azdajic@kbcsm.hr

J. M. Brozić
Department of Oncology and Nuclear Medicine, Sestre Milosrdnice University Hospital Center, Zagreb, Croatia
e-mail: jasmina.maric.brozic@kbcsm.hr

A. Goren
Applied Biology, Inc., Irvine, CA, USA
e-mail: andyg@appliedbiology.com

5

T. Lotti et al. (eds.), *Clinical Cases in Melanoma*, Clinical Cases in Dermatology, https://doi.org/10.1007/978-3-030-50820-3_2

Fig. 2.1 (**a**, **b**) Widespread erythematous macules with pustular blistering on the trunk

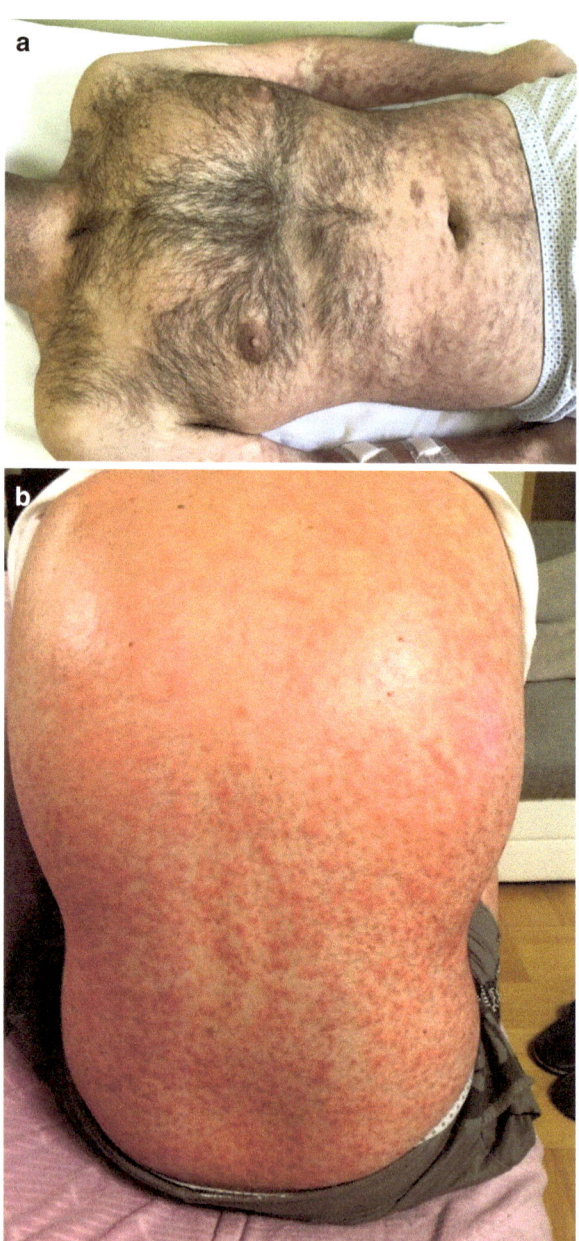

of systemic corticosteroids was prescribed and combined therapy was immediately stopped.

Based on the case description and the photographs, what is your diagnosis?

- Intraepithelial epithelioma
- Acute generalized exanthematic pustulosis

Fig. 2.2 Target lesions seen to be present on the extremities

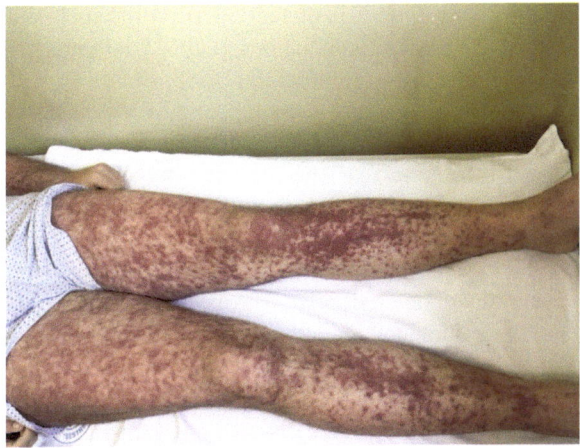

- Toxic shock syndrome
- Exfoliative dermatitis
- Toxic epidermal necrolysis

The cutaneous target lesions continued to spread on the face, trunk, and extremities, with palmoplantar involvement, revealing clear clinical picture of toxic epidermal necrolysis (Fig. 2.2), covering more than 80% of total body surface area, with mucosal erosions and whitish deposits in buccal area together with positive Nikolsky's sign. The skin changes were followed by fevers, chills, bone pain and elevated inflammatory parameters (Erythrocyte Sedimentation Rate 27 mm/3.6 ks, C-reactive protein 153.3 mg/L). The patient was treated with supportive measures and local corticosteroid therapy, while systemic corticosteroid therapy was discontinued due to lack of efficacy. Over the next few days the patient experienced regression of skin eruption and normalization of laboratory parameters. The patient was discharged after 1 week without further skin complications, but in following months the initial disease progressed and he died of multi-organ failure.

Diagnosis

Toxic epidermal necrolysis.

Discussion

Approximately 50% of all patients with cutaneous melanomas have tumours with an activating *BRAF* mutation [1]. The development of inhibitors of activated *BRAF* represents an important therapeutic option in cases of metastatic melanoma that contains the characteristic active *BRAF* mutation. Vemurafenib is a potent inhibitor of the kinase domain in mutant *BRAF*, while cobimetinib is a highly selective inhibitor of *MEK* [2]. Combinations of *BRAF* inhibitors and *MEK* inhibitors have been associated with more durable response rate [3], and they are commonly used as combined target therapy among patients with metastatic melanoma. However, previous studies have shown that combined target therapy commonly causes wide spectrum of adverse events [4]. Majority of these reactions in combined therapy are mild to moderate [5], therefore, they are common therapeutical option for oncological patients.

Severe adverse events to combined therapy such as Stevens-Johnson syndrome/toxic epidermal necrolysis have been reported rarely; more frequent if previous immunotherapy has been conducted in the treatment of metastatic melanoma. Our patient is a rare case of toxic epidermal necrolysis associated with the combination of targeted therapy (vemurafenib plus cobimetinib). This case confirms the importance of early recognition, monitoring and appropriate management that are all essential therapeutic steps in the treatment of severe adverse reactions caused by combined therapy.

Key Points

- Combined target therapy commonly causes mild to moderate adverse events on the skin (such as rash, hyperkeratosis and photosensitivity reaction).
- Serious adverse events such as Stevens-Johnson syndrome and toxic epidermal necrolysis induced by combined therapy are rare, but life-threating conditions and should be recognized and treated on time.

References

1. Ascierto PA, Kirkwood JM, Grob JJ, Simeone E, Grimaldi AM, Maio M, et al. The role of BRAF V600 mutation in melanoma. J Transl Med. 2012;10:85.
2. Sanchez JN, Wang T, Cohen MS. BRAF and MEK inhibitors: use and resistance in BRAF-mutated cancers. Drugs. 2018;78(5):549–66.
3. Faghfuri E, Nikfar S, Niaz K, Faramarzi MA, Abdollahi M. Mitogen-activated protein kinase (MEK) inhibitors to treat melanoma alone or in combination with other kinase inhibitors. Expert Opin Drug Metab Toxicol. 2018;14:317–30.
4. Dréno B, Ribas A, Larkin J, Hauschild A, Thomas L, Grob JJ, et al. Incidence, course, and management of toxicities associated with cobimetinib in combination with vemurafenib in the coBRIM study. Ann Oncol. 2017;28:1137–44.
5. Ascierto PA, McArthur GA, Dréno B, Atkinson V, Liszkay G, Di Giacomo AM, et al. Cobimetinib combined with vemurafenib in advanced BRAF(V600)-mutant melanoma (coBRIM): updated efficacy results from a randomised, double-blind, phase 3 trial. Lancet Oncol. 2016;17:1248–60.

Chapter 3
Treatment of a Longitudinal Melanonychia in One Session with a 532 nm Picosecond Laser

K. Fritz, M. Alghamdi, and C. Salavastru

A Caucasian female patient, age 52 years, presented on her left thumb nail a longitudinal melanonychia, persisting since more than 3 years without involvement of the nail edges (negative Hutchinson sign) and without any symptoms of internal and genetic diseases or dermatoses of the nail bed.

Since Melanonychia caused by a serious disease doesn't typically fade, we decided to perform one single session of laser therapy using a picosecond laser (PicoCare, WonTech, Korea) at 350 ps pulse duration, 532 nm, fluence 0.5 J, spot-size: 3 mm, 2 Hz and a total of 72 shots. For additional pain reduction we used air cooling during and immediately after laser treatment. The treatment was very well tolerated and resulted in a 95% pigment reduction after this one single session without any damage of the nail and without side effects. The pigmentation did not occur within the following 8 months.

Based on the case description and the photograph, what is your diagnosis?

1. Benign genetic Melanonychia
2. Trauma and/or infection triggered melanonychia
3. Lichen planus of the nail
4. Subungual melanoma

K. Fritz (✉)
Dermatology and Laser Center, Landau in der Pfalz, Germany

Carol Davila University, Bucharest, Romania
e-mail: drklausfritz@drklausfritz.com

M. Alghamdi
Dermatology and Laser Center, Landau in der Pfalz, Germany

Department of Dermatology, Al Baha University, Al Baha, Saudi Arabia

C. Salavastru
Carol Davila University, Bucharest, Romania

© The Editor(s) (if applicable) and The Author(s), under exclusive license to Springer Nature Switzerland AG 2020
T. Lotti et al. (eds.), *Clinical Cases in Melanoma*,
Clinical Cases in Dermatology, https://doi.org/10.1007/978-3-030-50820-3_3

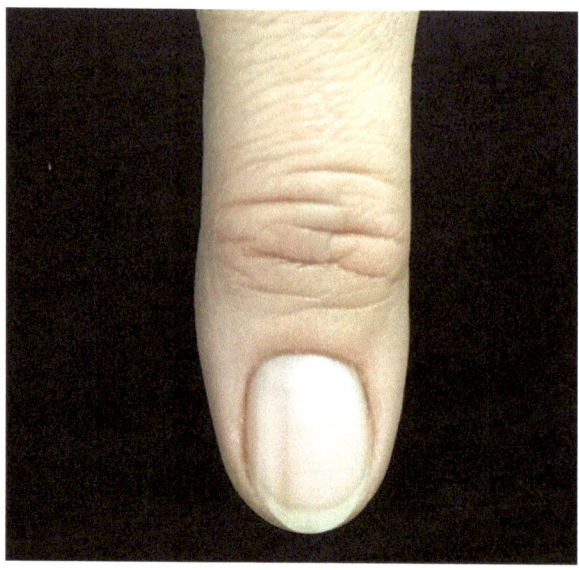

Melanonychia 0 before

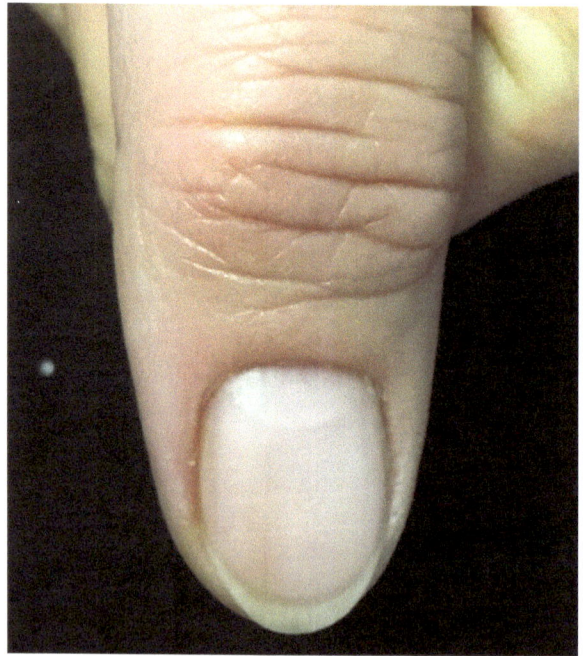

Melanonychia 1 post 1 day 1 session

Diagnosis

Benign acquired melanonychia (due to trauma or infection).

Melanonychia in this patient was due to nail invasion by melanin-producing pathogens. Our patient did not show the key symptom of subungual melanoma, the "Hutchinson's sign," a streak which extends from the tip of the nail all the way down to the nail bed and into the cuticle. She also did not show any signs of internal, genetic or immunologic diseases and due to the fact that the pigmentation faded without recurrence melanoma was most unlikely. So we decided not to biopsy the lesion.

Discussion

So far biopsies are the only way to differentiate between possible melanoma and other causes, this is why any additional and easy diagnostic or therapeutic approach is welcome. Temporary or less serious melanonychia disappears easily with laser treatment and in many cases does not reoccur or at least much less. This allows a clinical differentiation between malign or serious reasons of this condition which can occur frequently in darker skin types for many various reasons. Picosecond lasers destroy pigments photothermical and éven more photomechanical—chromophore independent—with better results than nanosecond lasers and less heat, which causes less pain during treatment on the sensitive nail plate [1].

Key Points

- The laser procedure helps in clinical differential diagnosis, which is not always sufficient and helps to avoid invasive surgical procedures.
- The laser treatment is effective, cosmetically satisfying, causes little pain and no down time.

Reference

1. Lorgeou A, Perilat Y, Gral N, Lagrange S, Lacour J-P, Passeron T. Comparison of two picosecond lasers to a nanosecond laser for treating tattoos: a prospective randomized study on 49 patients. J Eur Acad Dermatol Venereol. 2018;32(2):265–70.

Chapter 4
A Strange Enlargement of the Upper Lip

M. Kacheva, M. Kassini, M. Kadurina, Z. Demerdzhieva, and N. Tsankov

A 44-year-old female presented to the office complaining of rapidly growing nodular lesion on the upper lip for the past 6 months (Figs. 4.1 and 4.2). She denied any major medical history or systemic disease.

Based on the case description and the photograph, what is your diagnosis?

1. Basal cell carcinoma
2. Squamous cell carcinoma
3. Adenocarcinoma
4. Angiosarcoma
5. Adenoid cystic carcinoma

Fig. 4.1 A 44-year-old female presented complaining of rapidly growing nodular lesion on the upper lip for the past 6 months

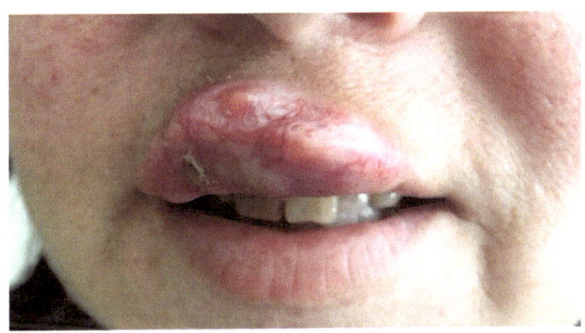

M. Kacheva · M. Kassini · M. Kadurina (✉) · Z. Demerdzhieva · N. Tsankov
Dermatology and Venerology Clinic, Acibadem City Clinic Tokuda Hospital,
Sofia, Bulgaria
e-mail: mira@kadurina.com

Fig. 4.2 Physical
examination revealed
5 × 6 cm enlargement of
the upper lip

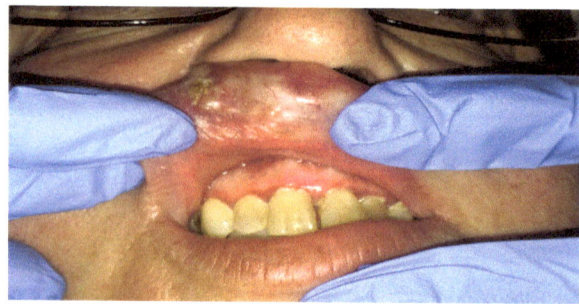

Fig. 4.3 Dermato-
scopic picture

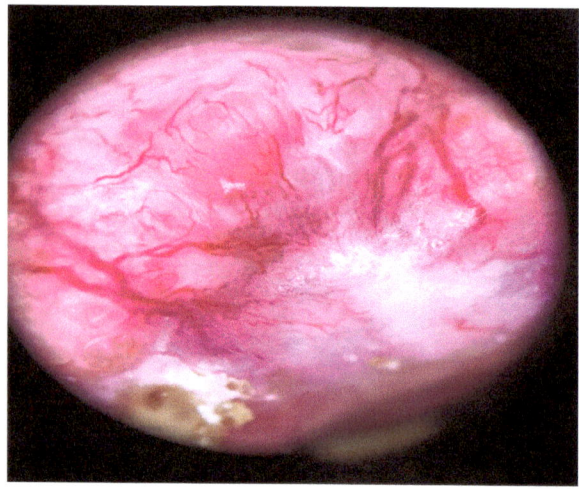

Physical examination revealed 5 × 6 cm. enlargement of the upper lip. The lesion
was erythematous with ill-defined borders.

Dermatoscopic evaluation showed polymorphous vascular pattern, multiple
shades of pink, milky red clods and white structureless areas (Fig. 4.3).

Biopsies for histopathological and imunohistochemical studies were obtained.
Microscopically nests and cords composed of pleomorphic or spindled cells lacking
pigmentation and showing basophilic nuclei, prominent nucleoli and frequent
mitotic figures, were scattered throughout the dermis (Fig. 4.4). Immunoreactivity
for S-100 and Melan-A was detected in the tumor cells (Figs. 4.5 and 4.6), but they
were negative for HMB 45 (Fig. 4.7).

Fig. 4.4 The tumor mass, infiltrating throughout the dermis; Hematoxylin and eosin stain

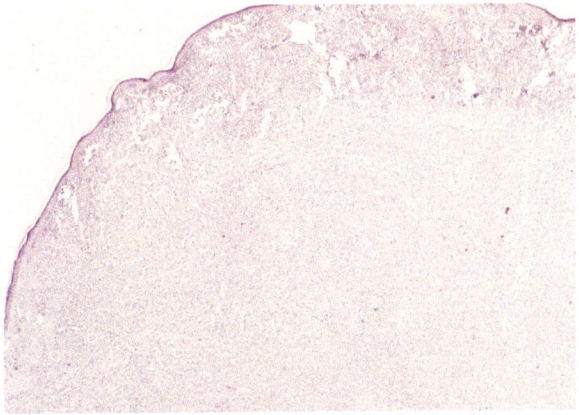

Fig. 4.5 The tumor cells showing positive immunohistochemical staining for S-100 protein

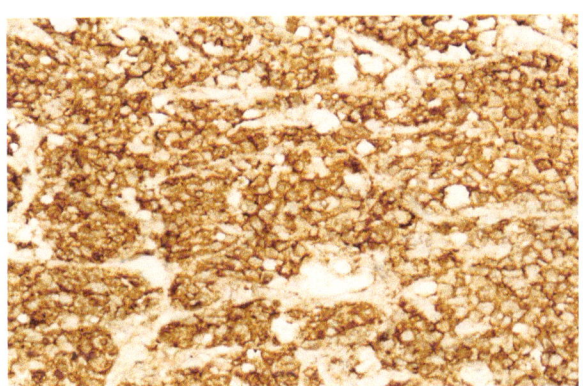

Fig. 4.6 The tumor cells showing positive immunohistochemical staining for Melan-A

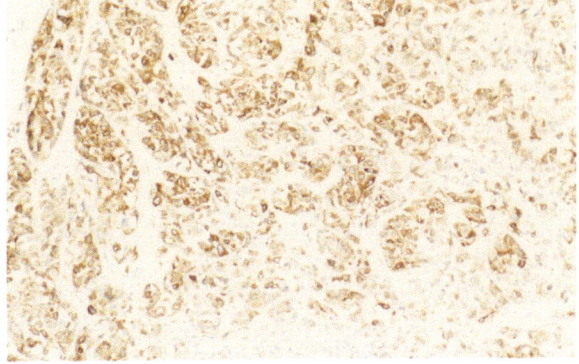

Fig. 4.7 The tumor cells showing negative immunohistochemical staining for HMB-45

Fig. 4.8 Clinical improvement after 6 courses of Pembrolizumab

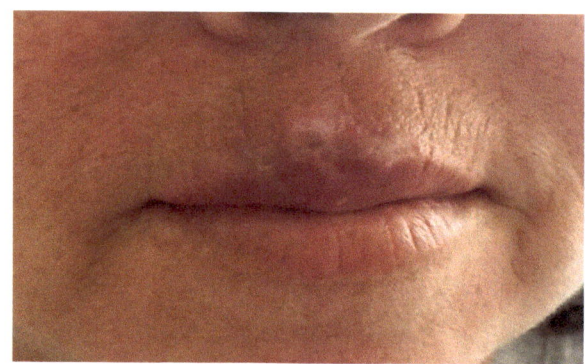

Diagnosis

Amelanotic Melanoma

Positron emission tomography scan showed malignant process in the upper lip and dissemination in three lymph nodes—two in the retromandibular region and one in the aortopulmonary window.

Magnetic resonance imaging of the head did not reveal any secondary changes of the brain tissue.

The BRAF V600 E mutation status was negative.

Based on the clinical, histopathological picture, specific localization of the tumor and the negative BRAF status, immunotherapy with anti-PD 1 monoclonal antibody (Pembrolizumab) was initiated at dose 2 mg/kg. Significant clinical improvement was observed after 6 courses of immunotherapy (Fig. 4.8).

Discussion

Amelanotic malignant melanoma is a subtype of cutaneous melanoma with little or no pigment on visual inspection. It may mimic benign and malignant variants of both melanocytic and nonmelanocytic lesions [1]. The incidence of amelanotic melanomas (AMs) has been estimated to be between 1.8 and 8.1% of all melanomas. Amelanotic malignant melanoma generally occurs on the trunk and lower extremities; it rarely is located on the lip with various clinical features. The diagnosis of AMM is a challenge for clinicians because it is a rare entity that presents with various clinical features [2].

Once AMM is diagnosed, treatment follows the same guidelines as pigmented melanomas [3]. However, AMM has a worse prognosis than pigmented melanomas, presumably because of the delay in diagnosis.

One key interaction between cancer cells and the immune system is mediated by programmed death ligand-1 (PD-L1) and programmed death 1 (PD-1) signaling. PD-1 is a member of the CD28 superfamily and is expressed on the surface of activated T-cells and B-cells.

Monoclonal antibodies against PD1 and its ligand (PD-L1), the second generation immunomodulatory antibodies, displayed significant durable benefits in patients with MM [4].

Key Points

1. Malignant melanoma is a neoplasm of melanocytes or a neoplasm of the cells that develop from melanocytes.
2. Amelanotic melanoma is a rare subtype of melanoma in which the malignant cells have little to no pigment.
3. Pembrolizumab is an anti-PD-1 monoclonal antibody which is effective for treatment of patients with advanced or unresectable melanoma.

References

1. Pizzichetta MA, Talamini R, Stanganeli I, et al. Amelanotic/hypomelanotic melanoma: clinical and dermoscopic features. Br J Dermatol. 2004;150:1117–24.
2. Park HC, Kang HS. An amelanotic malignant melanoma of the lip: unusual shape and atypical location. Cutis. 2013;92(5):250–2.
3. Adler MJ, White CR Jr. Amelanotic malignant melanoma. Semin Cutan Med Surg. 1997;16:122–30.
4. Lin Z, Chen X, Li Z, et al. PD-1 antibody monotherapy for malignant melanoma: a systematic review and meta-analysis. PLoS One. 2016;11(8):e0160485. https://doi.org/10.1371/journal.pone.0160485.

Chapter 5
Elderly Man with Nail Pigmentation and Destruction

E. Eid and Abdul-Ghani Kibbi

A 79-year-old man presents with a 2-year history of gradually enlarging and spatially fixed pigmentation in the center of the nail. Concomitant nail destruction was first noted 1 year ago. He does not recall any history of trauma to the involved nail prior to the current complaint. The patient denies any toe pain, suppuration, or other symptoms (Fig. 5.1).

On physical exam, the nail plate of the right toe is remarkably thin and fragile; furthermore, a hyperpigmented morphologically vague lesion is noted centrally underneath the nail plate with two small hyperpigmented macules on the hyponychium. The epithelium surrounding the nail plate is erythematous. The rest of the toenails on both feet exhibit yellow discoloration and mild thickening.

Based on the Case Description and the Photograph, What Is Your Diagnosis?

1. Chronic paronychia
2. Onychomycosis
3. Subungual hematoma
4. Acral lentiginous melanoma

E. Eid
Department of Dermatology, American University of Beirut Medical Center, Beirut, Lebanon

A.-G. Kibbi (✉)
Faculty Affairs, Faculty of Medicine, Department of Dermatology, Medical Staff Affairs, American University of Beirut, Beirut, Lebanon
e-mail: agkibbi@aub.edu.lb

T. Lotti et al. (eds.), *Clinical Cases in Melanoma*, Clinical Cases in Dermatology, https://doi.org/10.1007/978-3-030-50820-3_5

Fig. 5.1 Destruction of
the nail plate with
underlying
hyperpigmented lesion and
erythema of the
surrounding epithelium

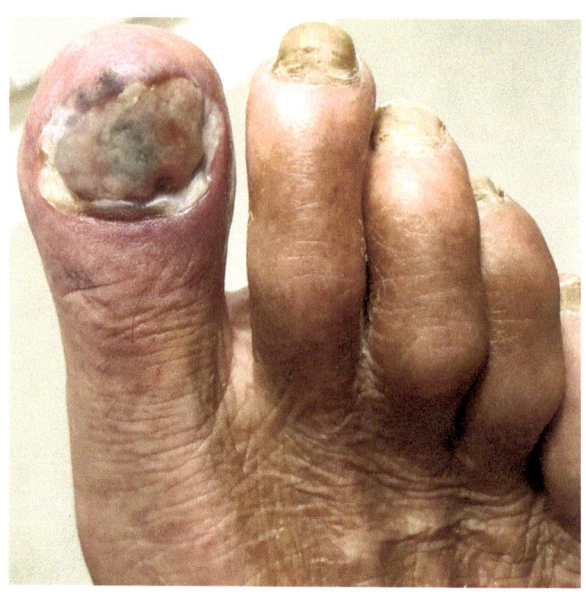

A punch biopsy of the central hyperpigmented lesion below the nail plate was obtained. Arising from a hyperplastic epithelium are individual as well as nests of atypical nevomelanocytes at the base of the rete ridges; moreover, similar cells can be seen extending as single units in a pagetoid manner. The cells are epithelioid and spindle-shaped and few contain melanin granules (Fig. 5.2a). The vertical growth phase revealed epithelioid and spindle shaped nevomelanocytes haphazardly arranged and of various sizes and shapes. Pigment laden macrophages are seen within the tumor cells and 4 in 10 mitotic figures per high power field were noted (Fig. 5.2b).

Immunohistochemical staining shows positivity for p16 and SOX10 and partial positivity for HMB-45. Ki 67 reveals a high proliferation index (Fig. 5.3).

Diagnosis

The diagnosis of invasive acral lentiginous (subungual) melanoma was made with a breslow thickness of at least 2.9 mm and a clark level of at least IV.

Discussion

On the spectrum encompassing the various clinical morphologies of cutaneous melanoma, subungual melanomas represent a notoriously difficult diagnostic challenge. Subungual melanomas comprise around 1.4% of all cutaneous melanomas [1] and

Fig. 5.2 (a) Radial growth: Nests of atypical nevomelanocytes aggregate at the base of the rete ridges. These cells are epithelioid and spindle-shaped and few contain melanin granules. (**b**) Vertical growth: Epithelioid and spindle shaped nevomelanocytes of various sizes and shapes are haphazardly arranged

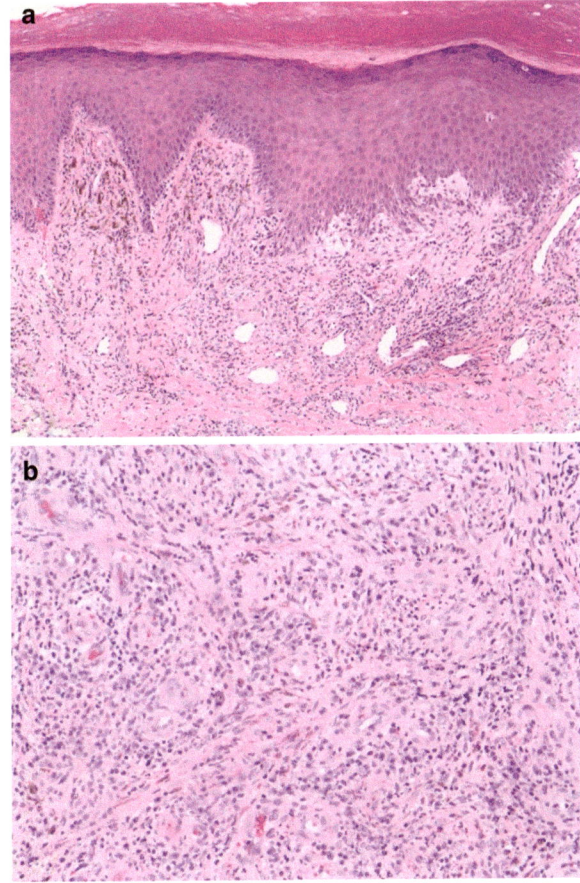

can manifest either as longitudinal dark bands on the nail (melanonychia) or as localized areas of nail hyperpigmentation as seen in our patient. Oftentimes, the hyperpigmentation of subungual melanoma characteristically transgresses the borders of the lateral and/or proximal nail fold leading to the melanoma-specific "Hutchinson's sign"; however, benign mimicry of the aforementioned sign, also known as pseudo-Hutchinson's sign, can present in several nail disorders such as nailbed melanocytic nevi and Bowen's disease of the nail further complicating early diagnosis of subungual melanoma. Later stages of subungual melanoma can present with ulceration as well as nail changes including elevation of the nailbed and nail dystrophy. As in all melanomas, histology is the definitive method of diagnosis and the subsequent elucidation of the radial and vertical growth phases are of paramount importance in prognostication and management. Immunohistochemical stains such as HMB-45, p16, and SOX10 are vital additional tools that increase the diagnostic capabilities by affording the dermatopathologist the ability to differentiate melanoma from histological mimickers. Rates of misdiagnosis as high as half of all cases of subungual melanomas have been reported [2]; the lack of physician exposure to

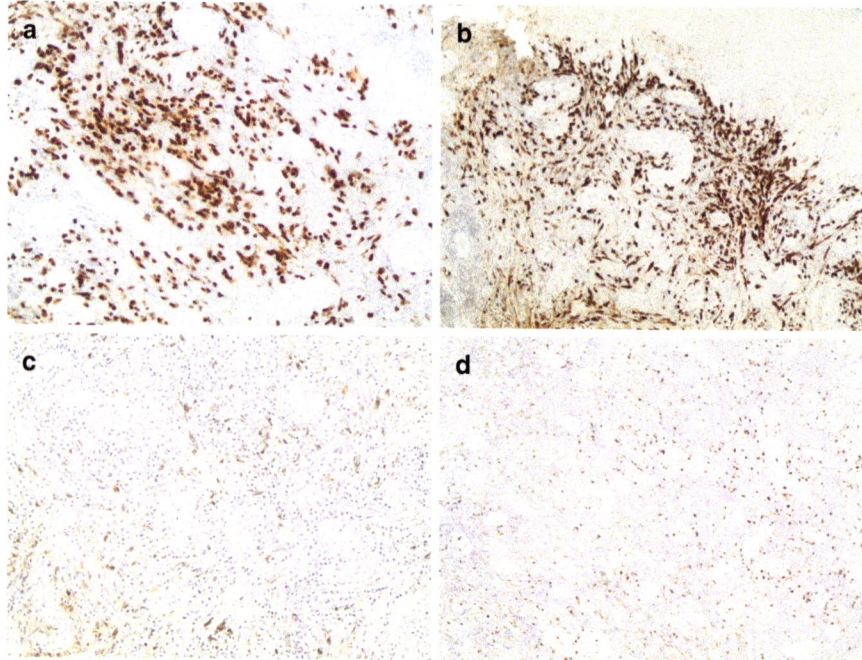

Fig. 5.3 Tumor cells positively stain for SOX10 (**a**) and p16 (**b**) and partially stain for HMB-45 (**c**). Ki 67 reveals a high proliferation index (**d**)

this entity in the nail locale secondary to rarity coupled with the absence of conformity to the "changing mole" pattern typical of many melanomas outside the nail have been incriminated as the main reasons. This high misdiagnosis rate coupled with a late patient presentation have subsequently resulted in a 5-year survival rate of only 51% [1].

Chronic paronychia is also worth mentioning as it can present with hyperpigmentation of the nail plate. This entity most commonly manifests secondary to a chronic infection of the proximal and/or distal nail fold or secondary to psoriatic or eczematous nail fold involvement. The subsequent retraction of the periungual tissue eventually results in nail changes such as nail dystrophy and onycholysis as well as discoloration of the nail. The latter can vary from green (Pseudomonal infection) to brown-black as seen in paronychia secondary to fungal infections (such as Candidal paronychia and Neoscytalidium paronychia among others) [3]; however, unlike our case, the discoloration is commonly located on the lateral distal edge of the nail.

In the elderly, onychomycosis, fungal infection of the nail, is a very common cause of nail dystrophy. It usually presents with thickening, onycholysis and yellow discoloration of the nail plate. Uncommonly, the onychomycotic toenail can adopt a brown-black discoloration especially when the invader is a pigment-producing non-dermatophytic fungus such as *Aspergillus niger* [4] or when a secondary bacterial infection by *Pseudomonas aeruginosa* takes place. In extreme cases, onychomycosis assumes a total dystrophic pattern whereby the affected nail witnesses a complete destruction of its nail plate.

A subungual hematoma commonly results from trauma to the nail damaging the subungual blood vessels. The resultant accumulation of blood beneath the nail plate may result in pain and secondary nail dystrophy. Alternatively, incorporation of an asymptomatic subungual hematoma into the ventral nail plate may occur on repeated microtraumas. In contrast to our case, a salient feature of subungual hematomas is distal migration mirroring nail growth. Dermoscopy is valuable in ascertaining the diagnosis as it allows the examiner to differentiate blood from melanin deposition; however, confusion can arise as hematomas can involve the cuticle and express the previously mentioned "pseudo-Hutchinson's sign".

Key Points

- Subungual melanomas can present as longitudinal dark bands on the nail plate or as localized areas of nail plate hyperpigmentation.
- Subungual melanomas can be easily confused with other benign entities; thus, the finding of nail plate destruction in the setting of nail plate hyperpigmented should alert the astute physician to the possibility of an underlying melanoma.

References

1. Banfield CC, Redburn JC, Dawber RP. The incidence and prognosis of nail apparatus melanoma. A retrospective study of 105 patients in four English regions. Br J Dermatol. 1998;139(2):276–9.
2. Metzger S, Ellwanger U, Stroebel W, Schiebel U, Rassner G, Fierlbeck G. Extent and consequences of physician delay in the diagnosis of acral melanoma. Melanoma Res. 1998;8(2):181–6.
3. Hay RJ, Baran R. Onychomycosis: a proposed revision of the clinical classification. J Am Acad Dermatol. 2011;65(6):1219–27.
4. Kim DM, Suh MK, Ha GY, Sohng SH. Fingernail onychomycosis due to *Aspergillus niger*. Ann Dermatol. 2012;24(4):459–63.

Chapter 6
A Lentiginous-Appearing Lesion on the Shoulder of a 49-Year-Old Caucasian Female with Intense Photodamage

Alejandro Martin-Gorgojo, Alicia Comunion-Artieda, Ana-Patricia Miguelez-Hernandez, and Francisco-Javier Bru-Gorraiz

A 49-year-old woman, with phototype I skin with no previous family or personal history of melanoma, presented to our department for a total skin check-up. The patient had numerous solar lentigines. Upon examination, a 9 × 4-mm brown irregular macule on the right deltoid region was detected. The dermoscopy showed apparent reticular pigmented pattern, along with some pigmented dots and a structureless central area with white-grey structures.

Based on the Case Description and the Photograph, What Is Your Diagnosis?

1. Solar lentigo
2. Seborrheic keratosis
3. Melanocytic nevus
4. Lentigo maligna
5. Melanoma in situ

A. Martin-Gorgojo (✉) · A. Comunion-Artieda · F.-J. Bru-Gorraiz
STI/Dermatology Department, Sección de Especialidades Médicas, Centro de Diagnóstico Médico, Madrid City Council, Madrid, Spain

A.-P. Miguelez-Hernandez
Dermatology Department, University Hospital La Princesa, Madrid, Spain

© The Editor(s) (if applicable) and The Author(s), under exclusive license to Springer Nature Switzerland AG 2020
T. Lotti et al. (eds.), *Clinical Cases in Melanoma*,
Clinical Cases in Dermatology, https://doi.org/10.1007/978-3-030-50820-3_6

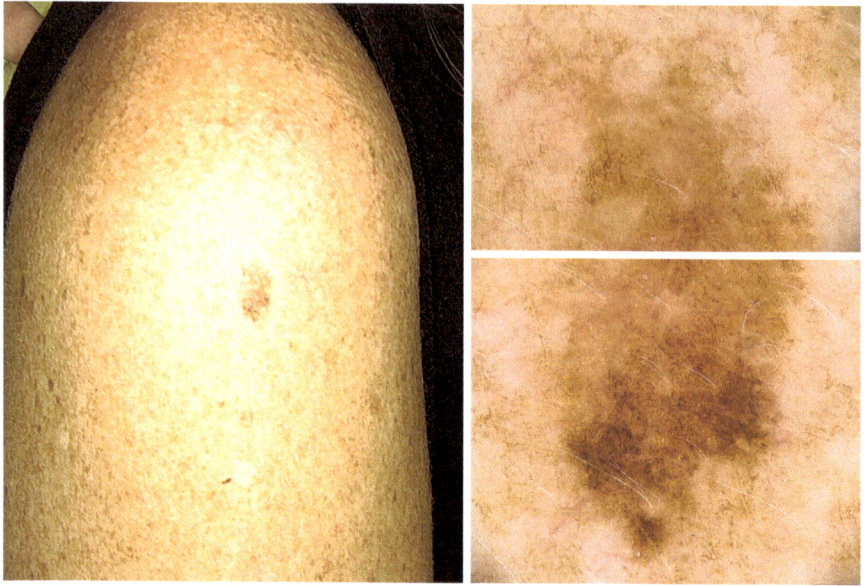

Left panel: Clinical presentation. Irregularly pigmented macule on the shoulder. Multiple solar lentigos on the surrounding skin.

Right panels: Dermoscopic image of the lesion (Fotofinder® dermoscope, 10×). The whole lesion couldn't be included in a single image, hence it is depicted in two panels.

An excisional biopsy was performed. Histopathological study showed atypical melanocytes with pagetoid epidermal extension, confined to the epidermis, and intense elastosis on the surrounding dermis.

Diagnosis

Melanoma in situ.

Follow-up

Upon diagnosis, 5-mm margins were excised. Two years after follow-up, the patient has shown no persistence or recurrence of the lesion and no additional melanomas have been detected to date.

Discussion

This case illustrates a melanoma in situ in a patient with intensely photodamaged skin. The histopathological diagnosis of these cases can be challenging: some authors have proposed that melanocytic density is the hallmark that leads to this diagnosis and aids to define the complete excision when the clinical or dermoscopic margins are not clear [1].

Although it was a lentiginous-appearing lesion and the diagnosis of lentigo maligna was considered [2], the histopathological appearance was clearly of a superficial-spreading melanoma in situ. This differential diagnosis is important and has its therapeutic and prognostic implications [3], which should be taken into account.

Finally, we believe this case can serve as an example of the 'ugly duckling' sign [4].

Key Points

- The 'ugly duckling' is a warning sign of melanoma. It refers to a pigmented lesion that stands out and looks different from the rest on the patient's skin.
- Melanoma that occurs on intensely photodamaged skin may pose some diagnostic and therapeutic challenges.

References

1. Speiser J, Tao J, Champlain A, Moy L, Janeczek M, Omman R, Mudaliar K, Tung R. Is melanocyte density our last hope? Comparison of histologic features of photodamaged skin and melanoma in situ after staged surgical excision with concurrent scouting biopsies. J Cutan Pathol. 2019;46:555–62.
2. Duarte AF, Sousa-Pinto B, Barros AM, Haneke E, Correia O. Lentigo maligna – not always a face and neck disease of the elderly. Dermatology. 2018;234:37–42.
3. Kunishige JH, Doan L, Brodland DG, Zitelli JA. Comparison of surgical margins for lentigo maligna versus melanoma in situ. J Am Acad Dermatol. 2019;81:204–12.
4. Grob JJ, Bonerandi JJ. The 'ugly duckling' sign: identification of the common characteristics of nevi in an individual as a basis for melanoma screening. Arch Dermatol. 1998;134:103–4.

Chapter 7
A Minute 'Ugly-Duckling' Pigmented Lesion on the Arm of a 60-Year-Old Caucasian Female

Alejandro Martin-Gorgojo, Alicia Comunion-Artieda, Angel Pizarro-Redondo, and Francisco-Javier Bru-Gorraiz

A 60-year-old woman, with phototype III skin and with no previous family or personal history of melanoma, presented to our department for a total skin check-up. One of his relatives, who was a physician, detected a 1-mm dark pigmented macule on the right arm that had been previously unnoticed by the patient. The patient had a moderate number of melanocytic nevi, predominantly macular. 10×-magnification dermoscopic imaging showed homogeneous pigmentation. 40×-magnification dermoscopic showed a central pigmented dark blotch, and surrounding pigmented dots and apparent peripheral streaks.

Based on the Case Description and the Photograph, What Is Your Diagnosis?

1. Lentigo simplex
2. Solar lentigo
3. Clark's nevus
4. Reed's nevus
5. Melanoma

An excisional biopsy was performed. Histopathological study showed atypical melanocytes with pagetoid epidermal extension, confined to the epidermis, with no other associated findings.

A. Martin-Gorgojo (✉) · A. Comunion-Artieda · F.-J. Bru-Gorraiz
STI/Dermatology Department, Sección de Especialidades Médicas, Centro de Diagnóstico Médico, Madrid City Council, Madrid, Spain

A. Pizarro-Redondo
Dermatology Department, Clínica Dermatológica Internacional, Madrid, Spain

© The Editor(s) (if applicable) and The Author(s), under exclusive license to Springer Nature Switzerland AG 2020
T. Lotti et al. (eds.), *Clinical Cases in Melanoma*,
Clinical Cases in Dermatology, https://doi.org/10.1007/978-3-030-50820-3_7

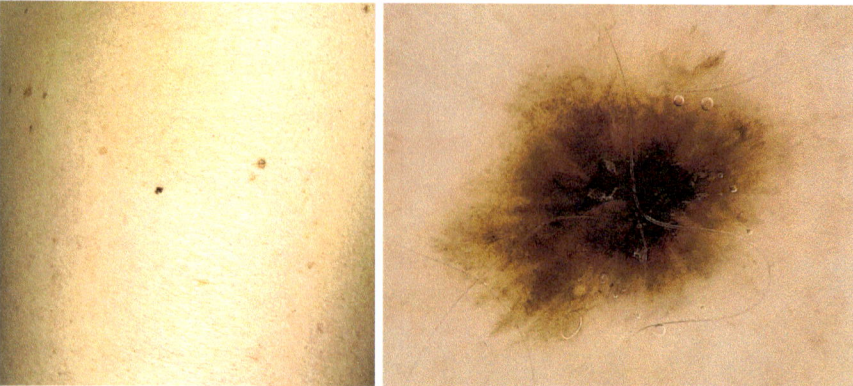

- Left panel: Clinical presentation. Minute darkly pigmented lesion on the lateral aspect of the right arm. Other lighter and equally small pigmented lesions on the surrounding skin.
- Right panel: Dermoscopic image of the lesion (Fotofinder® dermoscope, 40×).

Diagnosis

Superficial-spreading melanoma in situ.

Follow-up

Upon diagnosis, 5-mm margins were excised. One year after follow-up, the patient has shown no persistence or recurrence of the lesion and no additional atypical pigmented lesions have been detected to date.

Discussion

This case highlights the importance of listening to the patients' (and their relatives') concerns regarding the appearance or changes of certain lesions, albeit being inconspicuous on a first glance [1].

It is also an illustrative case of the 'ugly duckling' sign [2] (the patient had no similar lesion upon total skin examination), along with the modified ABCDE criteria (being a darkly pigmented lesion) [3] and of a small-diameter melanoma (or 'micro-melanoma'). Small-diameter melanomas are defined by a maximum clinical diameter of ≤6 mm (although some series have proposed a maximum diameter of

≤3 mm) [4–6]. Though the long-term biological behavior of these very small or incipient lesions is uncertain, proper excision is currently considered the most appropriate therapeutic approach [7].

Finally, we believe that the case gives us the opportunity to consider how we should modulate the messages that we give during a consultation (bearing in mind, too, when and whom should we give patients and their partners advice for, e.g., skin checkups and the features of concerning lesions) [8].

Key Points

- It is important to listen to the patients' (and their relatives') concerns regarding pigmented lesions, albeit being inconspicuous on a first glance.
- The 'ugly duckling' is a warning sign of melanoma. It refers to a pigmented lesion that stands out and looks different from the rest on the patient's skin.
- The modified ABCDE criteria is useful to detect small-diameter melanomas: in these cases, 'D' stands for 'Dark' pigmentation of a lesion.
- Although the long-term biological behavior of very small or incipient melanomas is uncertain, proper diagnosis and excision is currently considered the most appropriate approach.

References

1. Swetter SM, Layton CJ, Johnson TM, Brooks KR, Miller DR, Geller AC. Gender differences in melanoma awareness and detection practices between middle-aged and older men with melanoma and their female spouses. Arch Dermatol. 2009;145:488–90.
2. Grob JJ, Bonerandi JJ. The 'ugly duckling' sign: identification of the common characteristics of nevi in an individual as a basis for melanoma screening. Arch Dermatol. 1998;134:103–4.
3. Goldsmith SM. A unifying approach to the clinical diagnosis of melanoma including "D" for "Dark" in the ABCDE criteria. Dermatol Pract Concept. 2014;4(4):75–8.
4. Bono A, Tolomio E, Trincone S, Bartoli C, Tomatis S, Carbone A, Santinami M. Micromelanoma detection: a clinical study on 206 consecutive cases of pigmented skin lesions with a diameter < or = 3 mm. Br J Dermatol. 2006;155:570–3.
5. Fernandez EM, Helm KF. The diameter of melanomas. Dermatol Surg. 2004;30:1219–22.
6. de Giorgi V, Savarese I, Rossari S, et al. Features of small melanocytic lesions: does small mean benign? A clinical-dermoscopic study. Melanoma Res. 2012;22:252–6.
7. Carrera C, Palou J, Malvehy J, Segura S, Aguilera P, Salerni G, Lovatto L, Puig-Butillé J, Alós L, Puig S. Early stages of melanoma on the limbs of high-risk patients: clinical, dermoscopic, reflectance confocal microscopy and histopathological characterization for improved recognition. Acta Derm Venereol. 2011;91:137–46.
8. Robinson JK, Mallett KA, Turrisi R, Stapleton J. Engaging patients and their partners in preventive health behaviors: the physician factor. Arch Dermatol. 2009;145:469–73.

Chapter 8
When Dermoscopy Exonerates a Suspect, and "Indicts" Another Lesion

Lawrence Chukwudi Nwabudike, Alin Laurentiu Tatu, Ana Maria Oproiu, and Mariana Costache

A 51-year old patient suffering from long-standing type 2 diabetes mellitus presented with a dark lesion on his forehead that had been growing for several weeks (Fig. 8.1). He had had a similar lesion several years before that had been diagnosed and treated topically as a seborrheic keratosis. Clinical examination showed a brown-grey lesion with clear but irregular margins and a smooth surface covered by few pits. The clinical diagnosis of seborrheic keratosis was confirmed by dermoscopy.

However, the attending dermatologist noted a tiny, approximately 3 × 2 mm, dark brown macule lateral to his left orbit (Fig. 8.2a). On further questioning, the patient revealed that the spot had been first noticed 4 years earlier, after a post-traumatic contusion had healed. Dermoscopy (Fig. 8.2b) showed multiple, white, featureless areas throughout the lesion, with dots around the periphery and clods in its central area.

L. C. Nwabudike (✉)
N. Paulescu Institute, Bucharest, Romania

A. L. Tatu
Faculty of Medicine and Pharmacy/Clinical Department, Dermatology, Medical and Pharmaceutical Research Unit, Competitive, Interdisciplinary Research Integrated Platform "Dunărea de Jos", ReForm-UDJG "Dunărea de Jos" University, Infectious Diseases Clinical Hospital "St. Parascheva", Dermatalogy, Galati, Romania

A. M. Oproiu
Carol Davila University of Medicine and Pharmacy, Bucharest, Romania

Department of Plastic Surgery, Municipal University Hospital, Bucharest, Romania

M. Costache
Carol Davila University of Medicine and Pharmacy, Bucharest, Romania

Department of Histopathology, Municipal University Hospital, Bucharest, Romania

© The Editor(s) (if applicable) and The Author(s), under exclusive license to Springer Nature Switzerland AG 2020
T. Lotti et al. (eds.), *Clinical Cases in Melanoma*,
Clinical Cases in Dermatology, https://doi.org/10.1007/978-3-030-50820-3_8

33

Fig. 8.1 Brown-grey lesion with clear but irregular margins and smooth surface dotted with pits

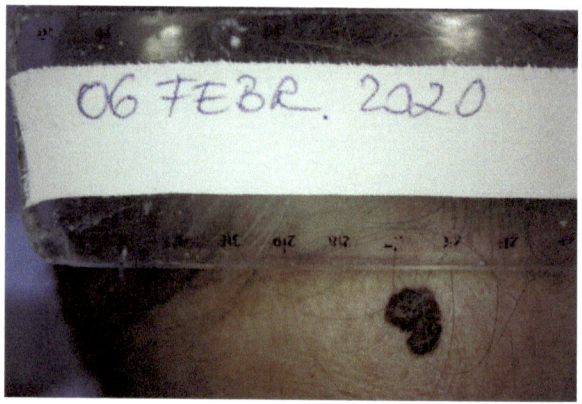

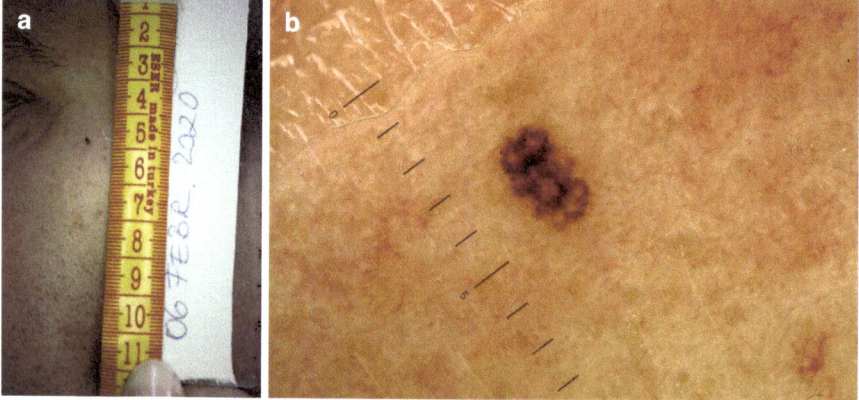

Fig. 8.2 (**a**) Small dark-brown macule lateral to the left orbit. (**b**) Multiple, white, featureless areas throughout the lesion, with dots around the periphery and clods in its central area

Based on the Case Description and the Photograph, What Is Your Diagnosis?

- Pigmented nevus
- Clark's nevus
- Solar lentigo
- Malignant melanoma

Diagnosis

Malignant melanoma

Discussion

The clinical diagnosis of melanoma was made and the patient referred for surgery.

Malignant melanoma is a malignant proliferation of melanocytes and there are three forms of melanoma, classified according to site—cutaneous malignant melanoma, mucosal malignant melanoma and uveal malignant melanoma [1]. Cutaneous malignant melanoma accounts for over 90% of cases of malignant melanoma [1] and is the 19th most common form of cancer worldwide [2], with an incidence of 197/100,000 in 2008 [2].

Patient self-discovery of a potential melanoma is more common than physician diagnosis (41.7% vs. 29.9% of cases) [3]. There was an average of 5 months delay between discovery of a lesion and reporting this lesion to the physician [3]. This delay period was over 4 years in our case as the patient considered the lesion benign. Of patients with delay, 43.2% felt the lesion was benign [3], whereas only 1.4% and 2% delayed reporting due to fear of the diagnosis and anatomical site [3].

Our case fits the literature pattern cited and underlines why it is necessary to continue to educate the general public about the potential significance of newly appearing pigmented lesions on the skin. It also shows the importance of a thorough skin examination by the attending physician, even for benign lesions.

Key Points

1. It is important to examine a patient for other pigmented lesions, even if the presenting lesion is benign.
2. Dermoscopy is an excellent and indispensable tool for triaging and diagnosing pigmented lesions.
3. A significant number of melanoma diagnoses are made by patients, so their concerns must always be taken seriously.
4. Better education of the public regarding significance of pigmented lesions is required so as to prevent delays in presentation.

References

1. Ali Z, Yousaf N, Larkin J. Melanoma epidemiology, biology and prognosis. EJC Suppl. 2013;11(2):81–91. https://doi.org/10.1016/j.ejcsup.2013.07.012.
2. Ferlay J, Shin H-R, Bray F, Forman D, Mathers C, Parkin DM. Estimates of worldwide burden of cancer in 2008: GLOBOCAN 2008. Int J Cancer. 2010;127:2893–917. https://doi.org/10.1002/ijc.25516.
3. Xavier MH, Drummond-Lage AP, Baeta C, Rocha L, Almeida AM, Wainstein AJ. Delay in cutaneous melanoma diagnosis: sequence analyses from suspicion to diagnosis in 211 patients. Medicine (Baltimore). 2016;95(31):e4396. https://doi.org/10.1097/MD.0000000000004396.

Chapter 9
A Growing Mass in the Left Foot

Sonia Sofía Ocampo-Garza and Jorge Ocampo-Candiani

A 54-year-old man with no relevant medical history presented to our dermatology clinic complaining of a growing mass in his left foot. He referenced a 4-year evolution with a small black "nevus". One year before the consultation, the lesion started growing, with occasional bleeding and pain. The patient had lost 7 kg of non-intentional body weight during the last 3 months.

Based on the Case Description and the Photograph, What Is Your Diagnosis?

1. Pigmented basal cell carcinoma
2. Kaposi sarcoma
3. Acral lentiginous melanoma
4. Subungual hematoma
5. Acral nevus

Upon physical examination, no adenopathy was found. An incisional biopsy was taken showing a melanocytic tumor with atypical melanocytes, mitotic figures (25 figures per cm^2), ulceration and perineural invasion. No angiolymphatic invasion, regression, or inflammatory infiltrate was present.

S. S. Ocampo-Garza · J. Ocampo-Candiani (✉)
Universidad Autónoma de Nuevo León, Department of Dermatology,
Hospital Universitario "Dr José Eleuterio González", Monterrey, Nuevo León, Mexico

© The Editor(s) (if applicable) and The Author(s), under exclusive license to
Springer Nature Switzerland AG 2020
T. Lotti et al. (eds.), *Clinical Cases in Melanoma*,
Clinical Cases in Dermatology, https://doi.org/10.1007/978-3-030-50820-3_9

Diagnosis

Acral lentiginous melanoma, Breslow 4.87 mm, Clark IV.

Discussion

Four major types of melanoma have been described: superficial spreading melanoma, nodular melanoma, lentigo maligna melanoma, and acral lentiginous melanoma.

Acral lentiginous melanoma (ALM) is relatively uncommon, accounting for 5% of all melanomas in the United States; however, among people of color (Hispanic, Asian, and African American individuals), it accounts for a greater proportion [1]. ALM typically develops in the palms, soles, or around the nail apparatus; presents as an asymmetric macule; brown to black in color, with irregular borders.

The diagnosis is based on clinical and dermoscopic suspicion and pathological confirmation. A history of change in color, size, or shape of a pigmented lesion can aid in the diagnosis. The major dermoscopic criteria for ALM include a parallel ridge pattern, characteristic linear pigmentation along the dermatoglyphic ridges, irregular diffuse pigmentation, a structureless pattern on a background of dark brown-black pigmentation, or the presence of conventional melanoma-associated structures (polymorphous blood vessels, ulceration, blue-black veil, and irregular dots or streaks in the periphery). Early detection is a key factor for survival [2].

ALM has a worse prognosis with a survival rate 10–20% lower than that of other types of melanoma. This may be due to the delayed detection and more aggressive biological behavior [1]. The strongest predictor of survival is tumor thickness or Breslow depth.

The primary treatment of ALM is surgical excision with an appropriate margin determined by the Breslow depth and sentinel lymph nodes in intermediate-thickness tumors. Advanced melanoma is generally treated medically with interferon, interleukin-2, and dacarbazine or with newer therapies: targeted therapy (BRAF and MEK inhibitors) or immunotherapy (CTLA-4, PD-1 inhibitors, and T-VEC) [3].

Basal cell carcinoma (BCC) is also a skin tumor and the most common human cancer [4]. It is a neoplasm of basal keratinocytes and generally arises within sun-damaged skin and rarely on the palms or soles. There are many subtypes of BCC, including superficial, nodular and infiltrating. All of the subtypes can be pigmented [5]. A helpful tool to differentiate pigmented BCC from melanoma is dermoscopy. BCC presents with some specific dermoscopic features, such as arborizing vessels, regular blue-gray ovoid nests and globules, and leaf-like and spoke wheel structures [6].

Kaposi sarcoma (KS) is worth mentioning in the differential diagnosis of this patient. It is a type of vascular sarcoma, with the etiologic agent being type 8 human herpesvirus. Four clinical variants have been described: classic, African endemic, iatrogenic, and AIDS-associated. The classic variant mainly affects the extremities of elderly patients and follows an indolent course; iatrogenic KS is found generally in posttransplant patients, and AIDS-associated KS is found in approximately 25% of HIV-positive patients. Lesions may be red-purple macules, patches, plaques, or tumors. KS can affect the skin, mucous surface, lymph nodes, gastrointestinal tract, lungs, or liver [7].

Subungual hematoma can mimic acral lentiginous melanomas. Hematomas occur after trauma, causing damage to subungual blood vessels. Blood accumulates under the nail plate. Acute hematomas are associated with pain and history of nail trauma. Subungual hematomas migrate distally as the nail grows, and the color ranges from purple-red to black. Dermoscopy is useful for differentiating melanin deposition from blood accumulation [5].

When melanomas are diagnosed at early stages, it can be difficult to differentiate them from acral nevi. Nevi have an indolent course; they are usually macular and display a uniform light-brown to dark-brown color [5]. Three classic dermoscopic features are associated with acral nevi: a parallel furrow pattern, lattice-like pattern, and fibrillar pattern [2].

Based on the patient's clinical history and physical and pathological examinations, the diagnosis of acral lentiginous melanoma was made. Transtibial amputation of the left leg and sentinel lymph node biopsy was performed, finding one positive node. The patient was lost to follow-up after refusing lymphadenectomy (Figs. 9.1, 9.2, 9.3, 9.4 and 9.5).

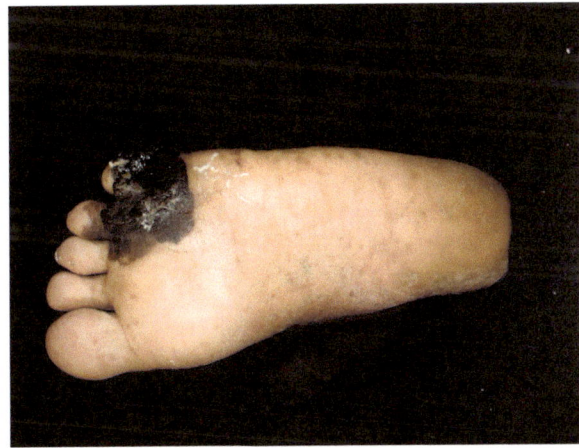

Fig. 9.1 Clinical image. Left foot with an ulcerated black mass involving the fourth and fifth toes and plantar region

Fig. 9.2 Clinical image.
Close up of the black mass

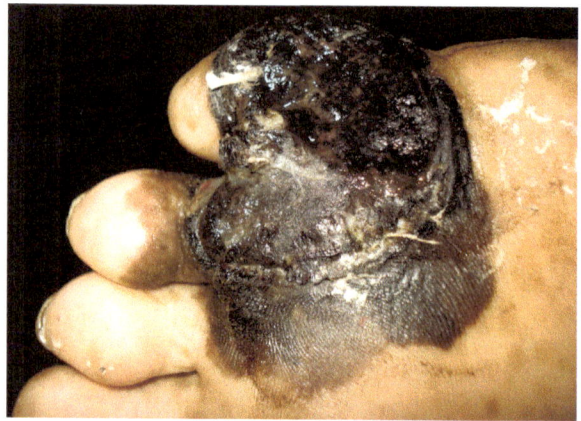

Fig. 9.3 Dermoscopy.
Parallel ridge pattern in
ALM with a structureless
pattern on a background of
black pigmentation

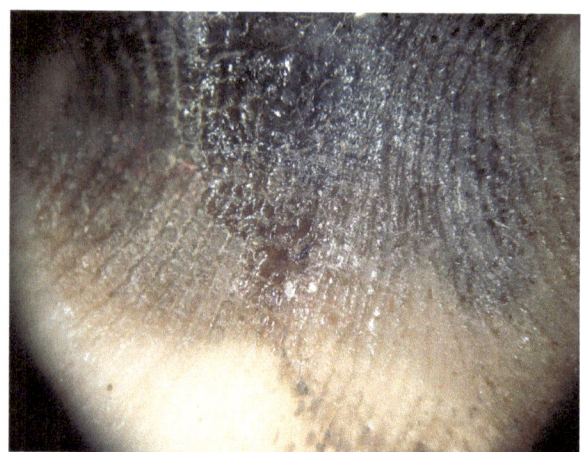

Fig. 9.4 H&E 10x.
Melanocytic tumor with
atypical melanocytes

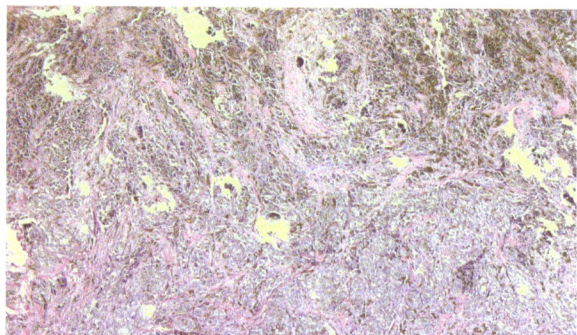

Fig. 9.5 H&E 10x. Melanoma with involvement of subcutaneous tissue

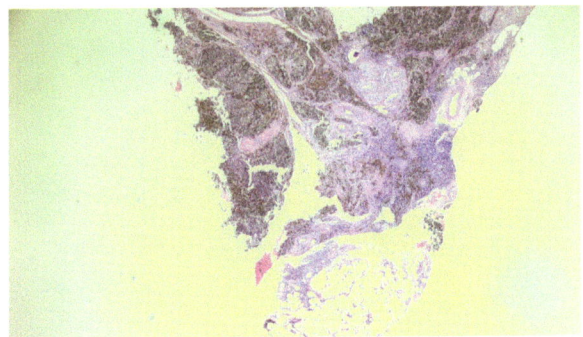

Key Points

- Acral lentiginous melanoma accounts for 5% of all melanomas, presenting as an asymmetric macule; it is brown to black in color, with irregular borders. It typically develops in the palms, soles, or around the nail apparatus.
- The typical histopathological features include asymmetrical proliferation of atypical melanocytes arising at the dermal-epidermal junction and invading the dermis. Pleomorphism, hyperchromatism, increased mitoses, and prominent nucleoli may be present.
- The standard therapy for primary ALM is wide local excision.

References

1. Asgari MM, Shen L, Sokil MM, Yeh I, Jorgenson E. Prognostic factors and survival in acral lentiginous melanoma. Br J Dermatol. 2017;177(2):428–35.
2. Tan A, Stein JA. Dermoscopic patterns of acral melanocytic lesions in skin of color. Cutis. 2019;103(5):274–6.
3. Swetter SM, Tsao H, Bichakjian CK, Curiel-Lewandrowski C, Elder DE, Gershenwald JE, et al. Guidelines of care for the management of primary cutaneous melanoma. J Am Acad Dermatol. 2019;80(1):208–50.
4. Bichakjian C, Armstrong A, Baum C, Bordeaux JS, Brown M, Busam KJ, et al. Guidelines of care for the management of basal cell carcinoma. J Am Acad Dermatol. 2018;78(3):540–59.
5. Bolognia JL, Schaffer JV, Cerroni L. Dermatology: Elsevier health sciences; 2017.
6. Reiter O, Mimouni I, Dusza S, Halpern AC, Leshem YA, Marghoob AA. Dermoscopic features of basal cell carcinoma and its subtypes: a systematic review. J Am Acad Dermatol. 2019;
7. Requena C, Alsina M, Morgado-Carrasco D, Cruz J, Sanmartin O, Serra-Guillen C, et al. Kaposi sarcoma and cutaneous angiosarcoma: guidelines for diagnosis and treatment. Actas Dermosifiliogr. 2018;109(10):878–87.

Chapter 10
Asymptomatic Longitudinal Band of Pigment in the Index Finger

Jorge Ocampo-Garza and Jorge Ocampo-Candiani

A 52-year-old female patient, with Fitzpatrick skin type III, presented with a 1-year history of an asymptomatic band of longitudinal melanonychia affecting her right index finger. Physical examination revealed a 2 mm band of longitudinal melanonychia with homogenous pigmentation in the central part of the right index finger (Fig. 10.1). Dermoscopy showed a 2 mm regular, homogenous band and the micro-Hutchinson sign (Fig. 10.2).

Fig. 10.1 Longitudinal 2 mm band of longitudinal melanonychia with homogenous pigmentation in the central part of the right index finger

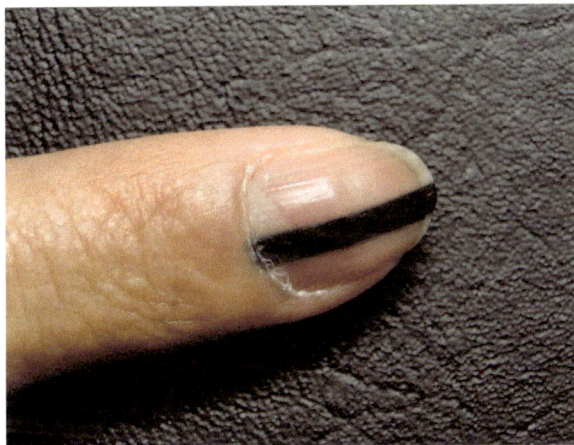

J. Ocampo-Garza · J. Ocampo-Candiani (✉)
Universidad Autónoma de Nuevo León, Department of Dermatology,
Hospital Universitario "Dr José Eleuterio González", Monterrey, Nuevo León, Mexico

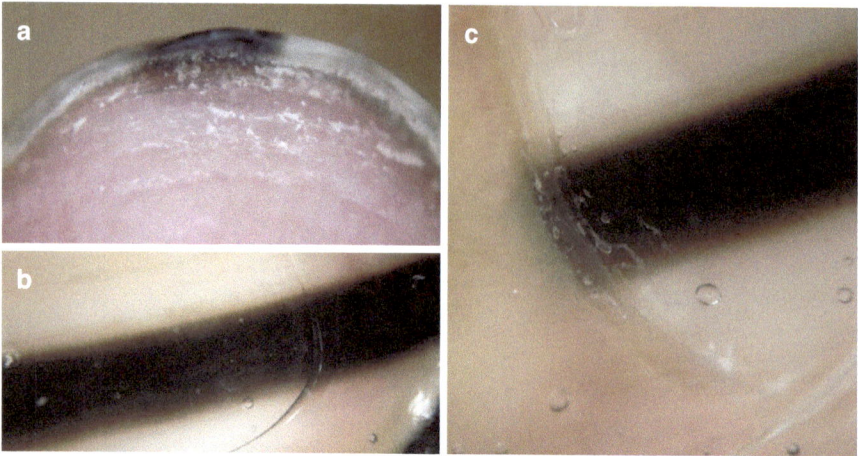

Fig. 10.2 Longitudinal melanonychia. Dermoscopy. (**a**) Free margin; (**b**) regular, homogenous band; (**c**) micro-Hutchinson sign

Based on the Case Description and the Photographs, What Is Your Diagnosis?

1. Onychomatricoma
2. Onychomycosis
3. Subungual melanoma
4. Subungual hematoma
5. Nail matrix nevi

A tangential biopsy of the entire pigmented band in the nail matrix was performed (reflecting the nail plate and allowing direct visualization of the band). Histopathology showed lentiginous proliferation of atypical melanocytes.

Diagnosis

Subungual melanoma in situ.

Discussion

Subungual melanoma (SUM) is an uncommon subtype of cutaneous melanoma that originates from the nail unit. The epidemiology of SUM varies among ethnicities, representing 0.7–3.5% of all malignant melanomas worldwide [1].

The etiology of the disease remains unclear. SUM typically presents as a pigmented longitudinal band with or without extension into the surrounding skin [2]. Levit et al. [3] proposed the ABCDEF rule for the clinical evaluation of SUM, where A stands for age (peak incidence in the fifth to seventh decade), African Americans, Asians, and Native Americans; B stands for the band breadth (3 mm or more), with brown-to-black coloration and variegated borders; C stands for change; D stands for the digit most commonly involved (thumb > hallux > index finger, single digit > multiple digits); E stands for the extension of the pigment in the proximal or lateral nailfold (Hutchinson sign); and F stands for a family or personal history of dysplastic nevus or melanoma. Other concerning signs of suspected SUM are a nonhomogenous pigmentation or triangular shape of the band, nail plate splitting, and blurred lateral borders [4].

Histopathological examination is still considered the gold standard for the diagnosis of SUM. The most important prognostic factor in SUM is the Breslow thickness at diagnosis. SUM frequently has a relatively poor prognosis compared with other types of melanoma because of a delay in the diagnosis [5].

The differential diagnosis of SUM includes hematoma, pyogenic granuloma, warts, callus, onychomycosis, squamous cell carcinoma, keratoacanthoma, foreign body granuloma, nevus, ingrown toenails, and several other nonpigmented cases [6].

Amputation was considered the treatment of choice; however, more conservative surgical treatments (wide excision) have been used in SUM in situ and in early invasive SUM with no difference concerning survival outcome but with superior results regarding functionality and cosmesis [7].

The patient had SUM in situ with a Breslow of 0.08 mm, and non-amputative wide local excision was performed, removing the entire nail unit with a lateral safety margin of 5 mm, followed by a skin graft (Fig. 10.3).

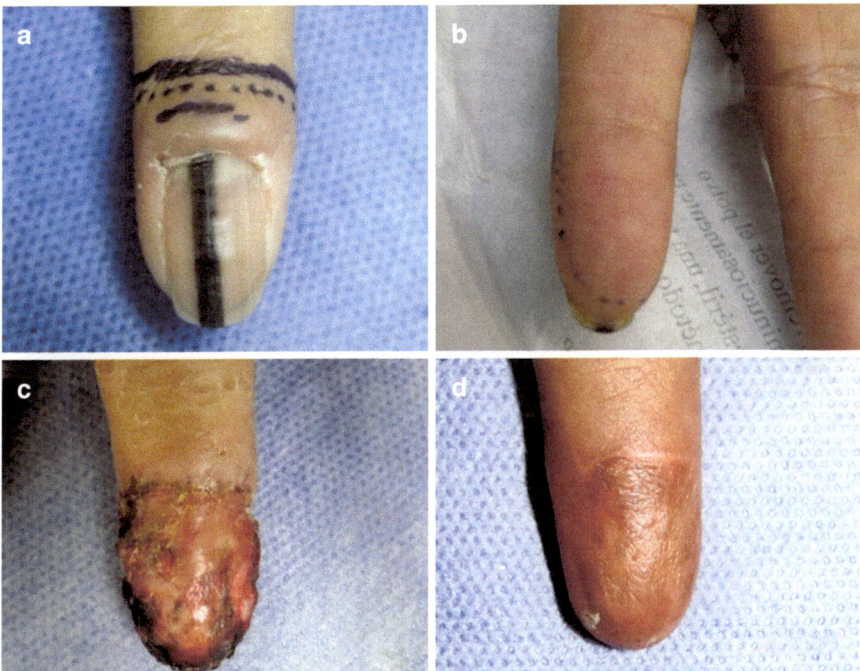

Fig. 10.3 Wide local excision. (**a**) Preoperative; (**b**) 5 mm margin; (**c**) 7 days after surgery; (**d**) at the 6-month follow-up

Key Points

- Subungual melanoma is an uncommon subtype of cutaneous melanoma.
- Usually presents as longitudinal melanonychia.
- Histopathological examination is still considered the gold standard for the diagnosis of SUM.
- Complete surgical excision is the treatment of choice for SUM.

References

1. Lieberherr S, Cazzaniga S, Haneke E, Hunger RE, Seyed Jafari SM. Melanoma of the nail apparatus: a systematic review and meta-analysis of current challenges and prognosis. J Eur Acad Dermatol Venereol. 2020;34:967–76.
2. Ocampo-Garza J, Gioia Di Chiacchio N, Haneke E, le Voci F, Paschoal FM. Subungual melanoma in situ treated with imiquimod 5% cream after conservative surgery recurrence. J Drugs Dermatol. 2017;16(3):268–70.
3. Levit EK, Kagen MH, Scher RK, Grossman M, Altman E. The ABC rule for clinical detection of subungual melanoma. J Am Acad Dermatol. 2000;42(2 Pt 1):269–74.
4. Ko D, Oromendia C, Scher R, Lipner SR. Retrospective single-center study evaluating clinical and dermoscopic features of longitudinal melanonychia, ABCDEF criteria, and risk of malignancy. J Am Acad Dermatol. 2019;80(5):1272–83.
5. Cochran AM, Buchanan PJ, Bueno RA Jr, Neumeister MW. Subungual melanoma: a review of current treatment. Plast Reconstr Surg. 2014;134(2):259–73.
6. Haneke E. Ungual melanoma - controversies in diagnosis and treatment. Dermatol Ther. 2012;25(6):510–24.
7. Duarte AF, Correia O, Barros AM, Ventura F, Haneke E. Nail melanoma in situ: clinical, dermoscopic, pathologic clues, and steps for minimally invasive treatment. Dermatol Surg. 2015;41(1):59–68.

Chapter 11
Clinical and Dermoscopic Simulators of Melanoma: Pigmented Bowen's Disease

André Laureano Oliveira and José Carlos Cardoso

A 40-year-old man, skin phototype II, was seen for a "mole check". He was not aware of a pigmented lesion on his right groin. A brown and asymmetrical macule with uneven borders and 1.2 cm of maximum diameter was observed (Fig. 11.1). Dermoscopy disclosed central hypopigmentation surrounded by multiple,

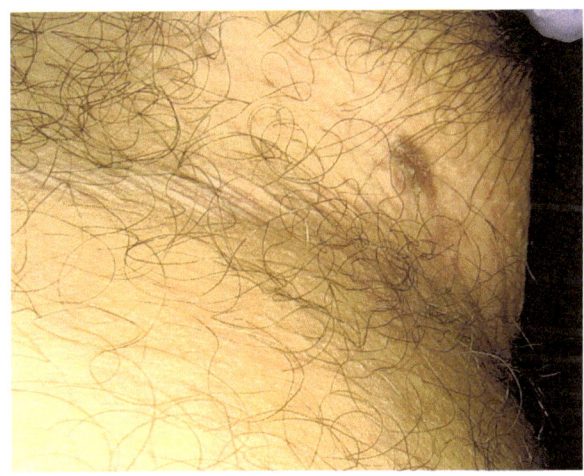

Fig. 11.1 Brown, irregular macule on the right groin, 1.2 cm in diameter

A. L. Oliveira (✉)
Department of Dermatology, Hospital CUF Descobertas, Lisbon, Portugal

Medical Faculty, University of Lisbon, Lisbon, Portugal

J. C. Cardoso
Department of Dermatology, Centro Hospitalar e Universitário de Coimbra, Coimbra, Portugal

T. Lotti et al. (eds.), *Clinical Cases in Melanoma*, Clinical Cases in Dermatology, https://doi.org/10.1007/978-3-030-50820-3_11

Fig. 11.2 Central white and pinkish structureless area surrounded by multiple, peripheral black dots with a linear fashion arrangement and structureless brown areas

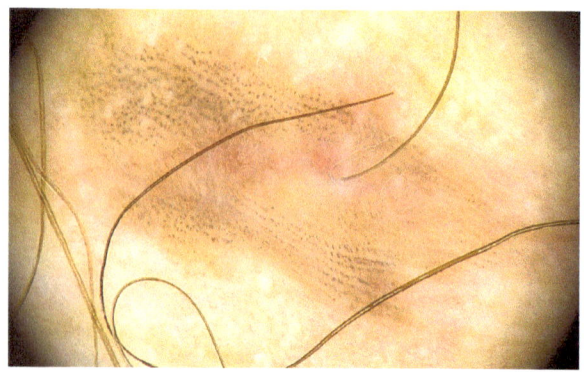

Fig. 11.3 Full-thickness epidermal cytologic atypia, suprabasal mitoses, melanin pigmentation in the basal layer and dermal melanophages (H&E x200)

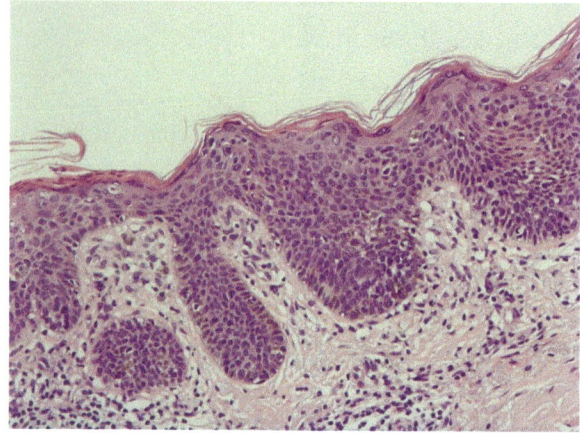

peripheral black dots with a linear fashion arrangement and confluent structureless brown areas (Fig. 11.2). After clinical and dermoscopic correlation the diagnoses of pigmented Bowen's disease versus melanoma were discussed. Surgical excision was performed. Histopathology revealed full-thickness cytologic atypia with acanthosis and confluent parakeratosis overlying a dysplastic epidermis with pleomorphic and dyskeratotic keratinocytes. Suprabasal mitoses, melanin pigmentation in the basal layer and dermal melanophages were also present, supporting the diagnosis of pigmented Bowen's disease (Fig. 11.3).

Based on the Case Description and the Photograph, What Is Your Diagnosis?

1. Melanoma
2. Seborrheic keratosis
3. Tinea nigra
4. Pigmented Bowen's disease

Diagnosis

Pigmented Bowen's disease.

Discussion

Pigmented Bowen's disease is a rare variant of squamous cell carcinoma in situ corresponding to about 2–5% of all cases [1]. Its presentation may simulate both benign, pre-malignant and malignant pigmented skin tumors, including solar lentigos, lichen planus-like keratosis, seborrheic keratosis; pigmented actinic keratosis; and melanoma and pigmented basal cell carcinoma; respectively. Pigmented Bowen's disease is also less common amongst patients with light skin types. Common dermoscopic features include a central white or pink structureless area (hypopigmentation), usually surrounded by black, blue or brown linearly arranged dots, confluent or multifocal black or brown structureless areas, network or streaks. In addition, glomerular or dotted vessels are also frequently seen within the lesion, associated or not with chrysalis under polarized light [2].

Key Points

- Clinical simulators of melanoma are common and include a wide variety of both benign or malignant, pigmented or nonpigmented tumors.
- Dermoscopic observation of peripheral, linearly arranged black dots was an important clue for the correct diagnosis of an otherwise rare presentation of Bowen's disease. Skin cancer is not always self-recognized by the patient. Be sure you make a complete skin inspection.

References

1. Zalaudek I, Argenziano G, Leinweber B, et al. Dermoscopy of Bowen's disease. Br J Dermatol. 2004;150(6):1112–6.
2. Cameron A, Rosendahl C, Tschandl P, et al. Dermatoscopy of pigmented Bowen's disease. J Am Acad Dermatol. 2010;62(4):597–604.

Chapter 12
Clinical and Dermoscopic Simulators of Melanoma: Dermatofibroma

André Laureano Oliveira and José Carlos Cardoso

A 52-year-old woman, skin phototype III, presented with a 6-month history of a rapidly-growing nodule on the left leg (Fig. 12.1). She denied any previous local trauma or insect bite, as well as history of skin cancer.

Clinical inspection revealed a brown patch with irregular and poorly defined borders, approximately 2.5 cm, with a 2 cm superimposed black and ulcerated nodule, while dermoscopy showed a central structureless pink and ulcerated area, surrounded by a yellowish area. There were also shiny white linear structures, areas of superficial brown crusts, polymorphous vessels and a peripheral pigment network (Fig. 12.2). The diagnosis of melanoma was considered. A fast-growing and ulcerated nodule corresponding to vertical growth from a superficial spreading melanoma (adjacent brown patch). The lesion was immediately excised.

Histologic examination revealed a nodular lesion occupying the entire dermis and hypodermis, relatively well circumscribed, and composed of spindle cells, histiocytic cells and multinucleated giant cells. There was xantomization and hemosiderin deposition in the histiocyte's cytoplasm (Fig. 12.3). A final diagnosis of a hemosiderotic dermatofibroma was made.

A. L. Oliveira (✉)
Department of Dermatology, Hospital CUF Descobertas, Lisbon, Portugal

Medical Faculty, University of Lisbon, Lisbon, Portugal

J. C. Cardoso
Department of Dermatology, Centro Hospitalar e Universitário de Coimbra, Coimbra, Portugal

T. Lotti et al. (eds.), *Clinical Cases in Melanoma*,
Clinical Cases in Dermatology, https://doi.org/10.1007/978-3-030-50820-3_12

51

Fig. 12.1 Brown plaque
on the left leg with
irregular borders, 2.5 cm of
maximum diameter,
underlying a 2 cm black
and ulcerated nodule

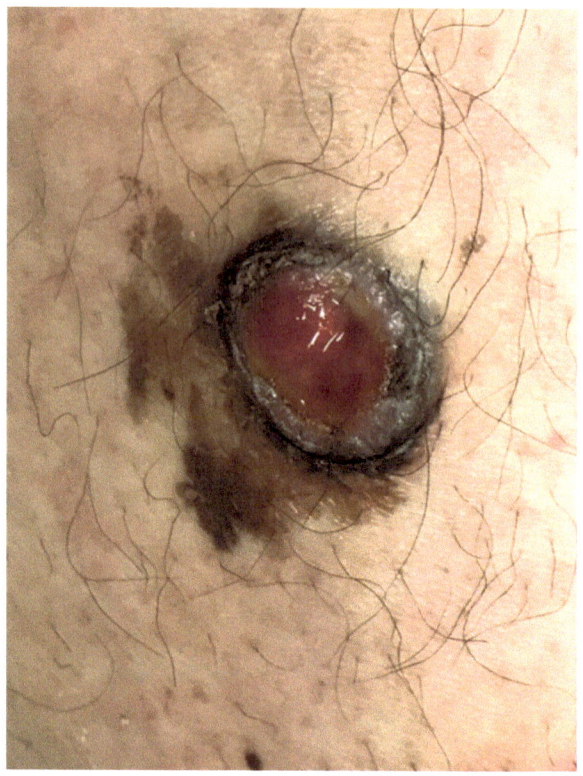

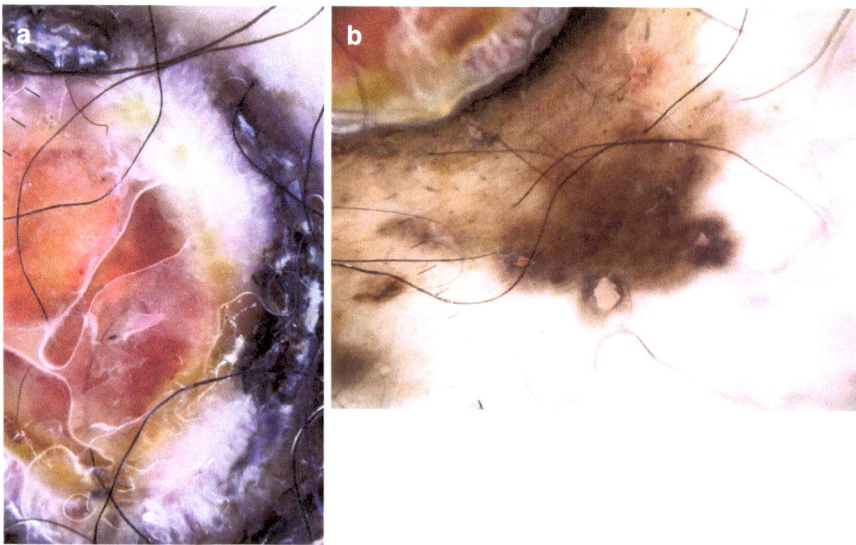

Fig. 12.2 (**a**) Central reddish and ulcerated homogenous area, surrounded by peripheral yellowish area; white linear structures, some areas of scale and irregular vessels, such as dotted vessels, can also be seen. (**b**) Peripheral pigment network

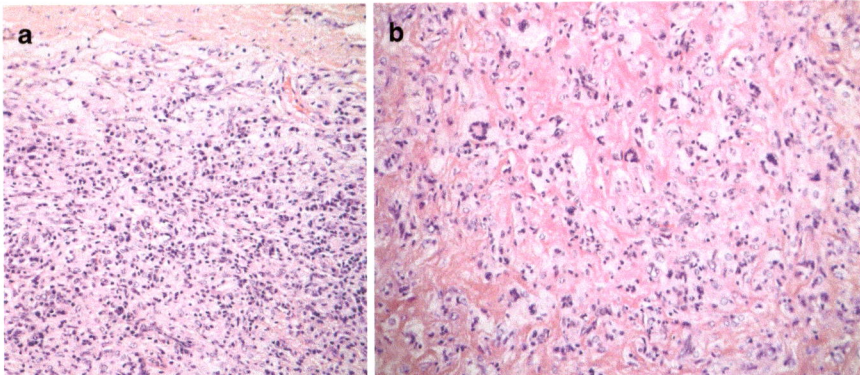

Fig. 12.3 Large nodular lesion that occupies the entire dermis and hypodermis, relatively well circumscribed, although not encapsulated, underlying a markedly irregular acanthotic epidermis. The lesion is composed of spindle cells, histiocytic cells and numerous multinucleated giant cells. There is extensive xantomization in the cytoplasm of histiocytic cells, some multinucleated giant cells, marked deposition of hemosiderin in the histiocyte's cytoplasm, and foci of hyalinization with more eosinophilic and amorphous collagen. (**a**: H&E x200; **b**: H&E x400)

Based on the Case Description and the Photograph, What Is Your Diagnosis?

1. Melanoma
2. Hemosiderotic dermatofibroma
3. Basal cell carcinoma

Diagnosis

Hemosiderotic dermatofibroma.

Discussion

Dermatofibromas might show a wide range of both clinical and dermoscopic presentation, sometimes being mistaken for other skin tumors [1]. Concerning hemosideric dermatofibroma, a significant association has been found with an atypical, melanoma-like dermoscopic pattern, which usually includes a central bluish/reddish homogenous area, corresponding to the prominent blood-filled spaces; white linear homogeneous structures, related to pronounced fibrosis within the dermis; a peripheral delicate pigment network, corresponding to hyperpigmented rete ridges; polymorphic vascular structures, associated with blood vessels in the stroma; a scaly surface, related to acanthosis and hyperkeratosis; and a yellowish homogeneous area at the periphery, associated with hemosiderin deposits or foamy giant cells which can be an important clue for this diagnosis [2]. Hemosiderotic dermatofibroma can therefore simulate malignant melanoma both clinically and dermoscopically, histopathological examination being essential for definitive diagnosis.

Key Points

- The complementary use of dermoscopy increases diagnostic accuracy, hence decreasing the need for unnecessary invasive procedures.
- A true diagnostic challenge was shown in the presented case of rare hemosiderotic dermatofibroma mimicking melanoma. Peripheral yellowish homogeneous structures observed under dermoscopy were an important clue for the diagnosis.

References

1. Kilinc Karaarslan I, Gencoglan G, Akalin T, Ozdemir F. Different dermoscopic faces of dermatofibromas. J Am Acad Dermatol. 2007;57(3):401–6.
2. Zaballos P, Llambrich A, Ara A, O Lazarán Z, Malvehy J, Puig S. Dermosccopic findings of haemosiderotic and aneurysmal dermatofibroma: report of six patients. Br J Dermatol. 2006;154(2):244–50.

Chapter 13
An Irregular Pigmented Lesion of the Lower Eyelid Margin

Asja Prohic and Suada Kuskunovic-Vlahovljak

A 74-year-old female patient presented to our clinic for dark brown irregular pigmented plaque in the area of the right eyelid margin. She gave history of a light brown macula in the same location since her young age. Over time, the lesion increased slightly and during the last year she reported progressive growth and color variegation.

On physical examination, 1 × 0.5 cm brown to black patch was found on the right inferior fornix and in the area of the right eyelid margin (Fig. 13.1).

Fig. 13.1 An elderly female presented with brown to black irregular patch on the right inferior fornix and in the area of the right eyelid margin

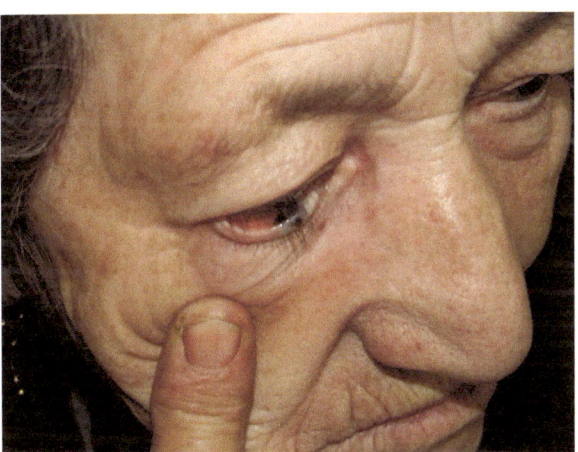

A. Prohic (✉)
Department of Dermatovenerology, University Clinical Center of Sarajevo, Sarajevo, Bosnia and Herzegovina

S. Kuskunovic-Vlahovljak
Institute for Pathology, Medical Faculty, University of Sarajevo, Sarajevo, Bosnia and Herzegovina

Based on the Case Description and the Photograph, What Is Your Diagnosis?

1. Melanocyte nevus
2. Nevus of Ota
3. Lentigo maligna
4. Malignant melanoma
5. Spitz nevus

Incisional biopsy from the margin of the right lower eyelid was obtained and histopathological examination revealed poorly circumscribed asymmetric lesion showing irregular lentiginous nested proliferation of atypical melanocytes exhibiting nuclear pleomorphism, pathologic mitoses ($1/mm^2$) and dusty melanin pigmentation. There were also foci of pagetoid spread. Atypical melanocytes were invading superficial parts of papillary dermis (Breslow thickness 0.35 mm, Clark level II). Immunohistochemistry showed HMB-45, Melan-A and S-100 positivity of atypical melanocytes.

Diagnosis

Superficial spreading melanoma

Discussion

Primary cutaneous melanomas of the eyelid are rare malignant tumors with an annual incidence of 0.6 per million whites over the age of 20 [1].

Despite its low frequency (less than 1% of eyelid malignancies and approximately 1% of all cutaneous melanomas), eyelid melanoma (EM) represents the most common primary nonbasal cell and nonsquamous cell malignancy of the eyelid [2].

There is no gender predilection, although some authors emphasize a slight female predominance. Mean age at diagnosis is about 68 years and more than a half of patients are older than 70 years of age [3].

Risk factors, as with other head and neck melanomas, include pale or freckle-dense skin, blond or red hair, and a positive history of at least two episodes of blistering sunburns by age 15 [3].

EM can arise from pre-existing nevus or de novo without history of precursor lesions.

In the majority of reported cases of EM, the lower eyelid is more commonly involved than the upper eyelid, as in this case probably due to its more direct exposure to UV light [3].

EM do not differ in clinical appearance than melanomas located elsewhere [4]. It typically appears as pigmented macula of the eyelid or extension of pigment from the conjunctiva.

As lesion enlarges, it may display color variegation, may be asymmetric, tends to have an irregular border and a diameter greater than 6 mm.

The most common histologic subtype is superficial spreading melanoma, followed by lentigo maligna melanoma and nodular melanoma [1].

EM that involve, or arise from conjunctiva, have a greater risk of metastasis, than eyelid melanomas that are strictly cutaneous.

The recommended treatment is complete surgical excision with a margin of 3 mm for EM of ≤1 mm in Breslow thickness or at least 5 mm of margin in excision of EM lesions >1 mm in Breslow thickness [4].

If surgery is not possible, local treatment with 5% imiquimod cream and radiotherapy can be used for lentigo maligna melanomas [5].

Key Points

- The most important findings raising the possibility of melanoma are: asymmetry in a pigmented lesion, color variegation, ill-defined or irregular border, diameter larger than 6 mm, and evolution over time.
- Early detection and complete surgical excision with tumor-free margins is "gold standard" for every melanoma of the eyelid.
- Patients with lower eyelid melanomas require close follow-up to prevent local recurrence.

References

1. Mancera N, Smalley KSM, Margo CE. Melanoma of the eyelid and periocular skin: histopathologic classification and molecular pathology. Surv Ophthalmol. 2019;64(3):272–88.
2. Lin MJ, Mar V, McLean C, et al. Diagnostic accuracy of malignant melanoma according to subtype. Australas J Dermatol. 2014;55:35–42.
3. Oliver JD, Boczar D, Sisti A, Huayllani MT, Restrepo DJ, Spaulding AC, et al. Eyelid melanoma in the United States: a national cancer database analysis. J Craniofac Surg. 2019;30(8):2412–5.
4. Harish V, Bond JS, Scolyer RA, Haydu LE, Saw RP, Quinn MJ, et al. Margins of excision and prognostic factors for cutaneous eyelid melanomas. J Plast Reconstr Aesthet Surg. 2013;66(8):1066–73.
5. Erickson C, Miller SJ. Treatment options in melanoma in situ: topical and radiation therapy, excision and Mohs surgery. Int J Dermatol. 2010;49:482–91.

Chapter 14
Dark Pigmented Ulceration on the Bottom of a Toe

Asja Prohic

A 66-year-old man presented with a non-healing, eroded plaque involving the bottom of a toe on the left foot, which started 6 years ago.

The lesion initially appeared as a dark pigmented, irregular macula, slowly enlarging and forming a plaque with ulceration.

Dermatological examination revealed an ulcerated black plaque measuring 2.8 cm by 2.0 cm.

Multiple foci of satellites discontinuous from the main lesion were noticed (Fig. 14.1).

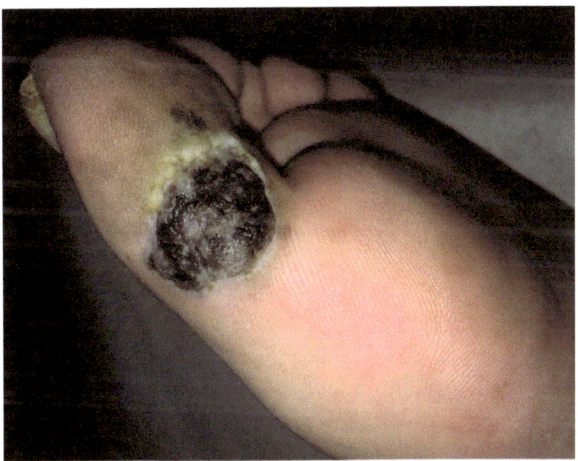

Fig. 14.1 Dark pigmented ulceration on the bottom of a toe

A. Prohic (✉)
Department of Dermatovenerology, University Clinical Center of Sarajevo, Sarajevo, Bosnia and Herzegovina

Based on the Case Description and the Photograph, What Is Your Diagnosis?

1. Non-healing arterial ulcer
2. Diabetic ulcer
3. Acral lentiginous nevus
4. Acral lentiginous melanoma
5. Pyogenic granuloma

Histopathology confirmed an acral lentiginous melanoma with a Breslow depth of 2.6 mm and immunohistochemical examination showed positive staining for melanoma associated antigens using the antibodies HMB-45, Melan-A and S100. A sentinel-lymph-node biopsy of the right inguinal nodes was negative.

After a multidisciplinary approach, a toe amputation and reconstruction of the local flap was performed using a skin envelope.

Diagnosis

Acral lentiginous melanoma

Discussion

Acral lentiginous melanoma (ALM) is a distinct subtype of melanoma most commonly found on the distal portions of the limbs. The term lentiginous refers to the histopathological pattern of melanocyte proliferation along the dermoepidermal junction, forming a sharp border between the dark skin and the lighter skin around it. This contrast in color is one of the most evident signs of this type of melanoma.

ALM is a very aggressive, malignant cutaneous tumor which usually reaches more advanced stages than other types of melanoma when diagnosed. The aggressive nature is reflected in a tendency to metastasize via the lymphogenic system and the hematogenic system to the visceral organs. Therefore, early recognition and treatment, consisting of excision in toto with clean margins, are essential.

ALM is the least common subtype of melanoma comprising less than 5% of all melanomas. However, it is the most common type of melanoma among Asians and dark-skinned individuals who are more likely to present with advanced-stage disease [1]. Among the white population, there is a predominance of women with the highest incidence in the seventh decade of life.

The occurrence and development of ALM is related to melanocytic nevi on fingers, toes, soles and on some specific areas where friction occurs. In addition, previous trauma, environmental factors, chemical stimulation, smoking and genetic factors have been reported to be risk factors for this subtype of melanoma [2]. Because ALM typically occurs in minimally sun-exposed areas, there is no evidence of overexposure to UV light as a risk factor of acral melanoma [3].

ALM occurs, as the name suggests, on the acral skin, most commonly on palmar, plantar, subungual, and occasionally, mucosal surfaces. Subungual variant of ALM typically occurs on the palms or soles or beneath the nail plate, most commonly on the fingernail.

A small percentage of superficial spreading and nodular melanoma may also occur on acral skin. However, numerous studies have found no significant difference in patients between ALM and other melanomas in the acral regions [4].

Lesions first present as dark brown to black pigmented macules or patches with irregular borders and variegated pigmentation usually larger than 3 cm in diameter. As the tumor enlarges it becomes papular, nodular or ulcerated, indicating deeper invasion in the dermis (vertical growth phase) [2, 4].

Immune-histochemical markers, S-100 protein and Human Melanoma Black (HMB)-45 are considered as sensitive markers in distinguishing between ALM and acral nevus [4].

Dermoscopic observations may help the diagnosis in the early stage of ALM. Irregular diffuse pigmentation and the parallel ridge pattern are the two most prevalent patterns.

Histologically, early-stage ALMs are characterized by diffuse proliferation of atypical melanocytes along the basal layer, with foci of confluent melanocytic growth. At the invasive stage, spindle or epithelioid cells extend into the papillary dermis during the radial growth phase [4].

ALM is melanoma with a poor prognosis, primarily because of its aggressive behaviour but also due to the fact that it is often diagnosed at an advanced stage than other subtypes of melanoma [1]. The clinical pathologic analysis, including Clark's levels and Breslow's thickness, are used to predict prognosis of ALM.

Wide local excision to achieve negative margins is the treatment of choice for all kinds of ALM [1]. In recent years, promising new treatments such as chemo immunotherapy, biologic therapy and targeted agents are improving survival rates for patients with melanoma [5].

Key Points

- Acral lentiginous melanoma is a rare subtype of melanoma on the acral skin surfaces, with plantar and subungual lesions being the most common sites.
- It presents as darkly pigmented macules or patches with raised areas and varying degrees of pigmentation and with ulcerations in advanced stages.
- Tumor is often diagnosed at later stages and the prognosis is worst among all types of cutaneous melanomas.

References

1. Goydos JS, Shoen SL. Acral lentiginous melanoma. Cancer Treat Res. 2016;167:321–9.
2. Jung HJ, Kweon SS, Lee JB, Lee SC, Yun SJ. A clinicopathologic analysis of 177 acral melanomas in koreans: relevance of spreading pattern and physical stress. JAMA Dermatol. 2013;149(11):1281–8.
3. Phan A, Touzet S, Dalle S, Ronger-Savlé S, Balme B, Thomas L. Acral lentiginous melanoma: a clinicoprognostic study of 126 cases. Br J Dermatol. 2006;155(3):561–9.
4. Li H, Liu X. Acral lentiginous melanoma. Clin Oncol. 2018;3:1548.
5. Nam KW, Bae YC, Nam SB, Kim JH, Kim HS, Choi YJ. Characteristics and treatment of cutaneous melanoma of the foot. Arch Plast Surg. 2016;43(1):59–65.

Chapter 15
Multiple Macules in a 40-Years-Old Female

Selma Poparic and Asja Prohic

A 40-year old female presented with a 3-month history of multiple, blue-grayish, thickly clustered, 1–3 mm in diameter macules increasing progressively in number and involving almost the whole left pectoral region. She revealed color change of a preexisting nevus on left areola, from light brown into black over the past two years (Fig. 15.1).

Dermoscopic appearance showed satellite nests of homogeneous melanocytic pigmentations with a blue nevus-like pattern. A presence of an oval, 5 mm in diameter, highly suspicious melanocytic lesion with areas of unstructured black, irregularly distributed pigment on the left areola has been detected.

Fig. 15.1 Female patient with multiple, blue-grayish, thickly clustered macules and color change of a preexisting nevus on left areola

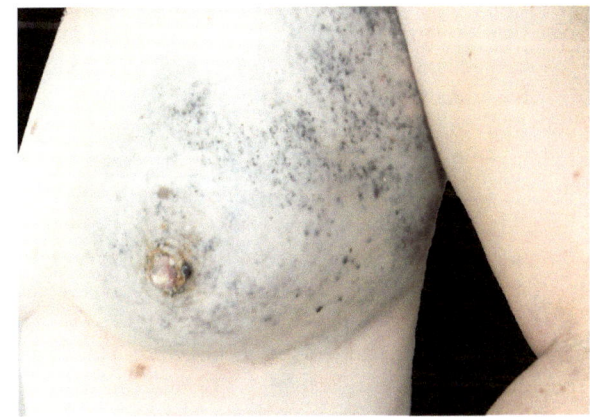

S. Poparic · A. Prohic (✉)
Department of Dermatovenerology, University Clinical Center of Sarajevo, Sarajevo, Bosnia and Herzegovina

© The Editor(s) (if applicable) and The Author(s), under exclusive license to Springer Nature Switzerland AG 2020
T. Lotti et al. (eds.), *Clinical Cases in Melanoma*, Clinical Cases in Dermatology, https://doi.org/10.1007/978-3-030-50820-3_15

Based on the Case Description and the Photograph, What Is Your Diagnosis?

1. Blue nevi
2. Nevus of Ito
3. Melanoma
4. Cutaneous metastases of melanoma
5. Breast cancer

Histopathological result and radical lymphadenectomy which showed axillary lymphatic invasion confirmed metastatic melanoma with positive staining for melanoma associated antigens using the antibodies S100 and HMB-45.

Diagnosis

Cutaneous metastases of melanoma

Discussion

Cutaneous metastases of malignant melanoma are defined as tumor lesions that can grow in any skin site over the regional lymph nodes. They are most frequently observed on the back in men and on the lower limbs in women, but can also occur in the same anatomic area of the primary melanoma.

Melanoma can metastasize by the lymphatic or by the hematogenous route as 'satellite' (up to 2 cm from the primary tumor), 'in-transit' (between the primary tumor and the regional lymph nodes) or 'distant' cutaneous metastases that appear in any skin site over the regional lymph nodes [1]. While the majority of cutaneous melanoma metastases have a known primary site, approximately 3.2% of them are presented in distant sites with no known primary lesion [2].

Common clinical presentations of cutaneous metastases include brown to black or skin colored macules, papules and nodules, which sometimes can ulcerate. Dermoscopic characteristics, which include whitish peripheral halo around a central blue area probably representing fibrosis, can be a valid diagnostic support, especially at an early stage of cutaneous metastases of malignant melanoma [3].

While the median survival is approximately 7 months for all patients with metastatic disease [4], the choice of treatment for cutaneous melanoma metastases depends on location and number of lesions, presence of systemic involvement, age and general health conditions of patients. Although the treatment is often palliative, new treatments such as cell therapy, gene therapy, and targeted therapy provide hope for the treatment of cutaneous recurrences of this most aggressive form of skin cancer.

Key Points

- Cutaneous metastases of malignant melanoma, are defined as tumor lesions that can grow in any skin site over the regional lymph nodes, mostly observed on the back in men and on the lower limbs in women, but can also occur in the same anatomic area of the primary melanoma.
- They are presented as brown to black or skin colored macules, papules and nodules, which sometimes can ulcerate.
- The median survival is approximately 7 months for all patients with metastatic melanoma, and, overall, treatment still remains unsatisfactory.

References

1. Garbe C, Peris K, Hauschild A, Saiag P, Middleton M, Spatz A, et al. Diagnosis and treatment of melanoma: European consensus-based interdisciplinary guideline. Eur J Cancer. 2010;46:270–83.
2. Kamposioras K, Pentheroudakis G, Pectasides D, Pavlidis N. Malignant melanoma of unknown primary site. To make the long story short. A systematic review of the literature. Crit Rev Oncol Hematol. 2011;78(2):112–26.
3. Rubegni P, Lamberti A, Mandato F, Perotti R, Fimiani M. Dermoscopic patternsof cutaneous melanoma metastases. Int J Dermatol. 2014;53(4):404–12.
4. Crosby T. Metastatic malignant melanoma. In: Hywell W, Bigby M, Diepgen T, Herxheimer A, Naldi L, Rzany B, editors. Evidence based dermatology. 1st ed. Prism books; 2003. p. 311–315.

Chapter 16
A Middle-Aged Woman with the 3-Year History of Nail Dyschromy

Aleksandra Opalińska and Adam Reich

A 55-year-old woman was admitted to the Department of Dermatology because of pigmented lesion within the nail plate of the fourth digit of the left hand. It was her first visit to a dermatology clinic, although the longitudinal melanonychia has persisted and grown slowly for about 3 years. She neither suffer from any chronic diseases nor report any additional subjective symptoms.

Physical examination revealed multi-coloured, pigmented lesion, about 4.5 mm wide, involving almost 50% of the nail plate (Fig. 16.1).

Based on the Case Description and the Photograph, What Is Your Diagnosis?

1. Subungual melanocytic nevus
2. Subungual melanoma
3. Subungual hematoma
4. Drug-induced longitudinal melanonychia
5. Pseudomonas nail infection

The dermoscopic view (Fig. 16.2) showed the following points:

- Multi-coloured, parallel strias, involving almost half of the nail plate
- Slightly trapezoidal shape of the lesion
- Minor dystrophy of the distal edge of the nail plate
- Pseudo-Hutchinson's sign.

A. Opalińska · A. Reich (✉)
Department of Dermatology, University of Rzeszow, Rzeszów, Poland

© The Editor(s) (if applicable) and The Author(s), under exclusive license to
Springer Nature Switzerland AG 2020
T. Lotti et al. (eds.), *Clinical Cases in Melanoma*,
Clinical Cases in Dermatology, https://doi.org/10.1007/978-3-030-50820-3_16

Fig. 16.1 Subungual
pigmented lesion within
the fourth digit of the
left hand

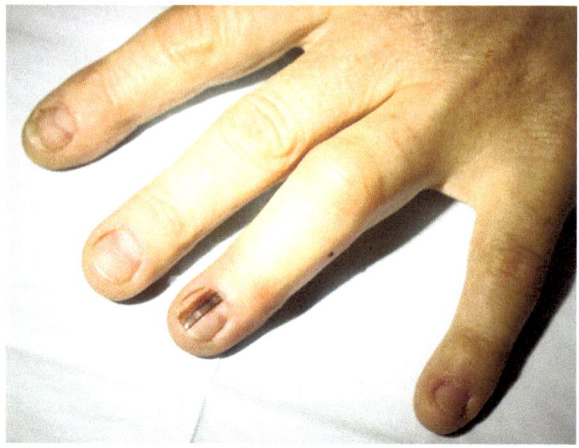

Fig. 16.2 Dermoscopic
view of the pigmented
lesion from Fig. 16.1

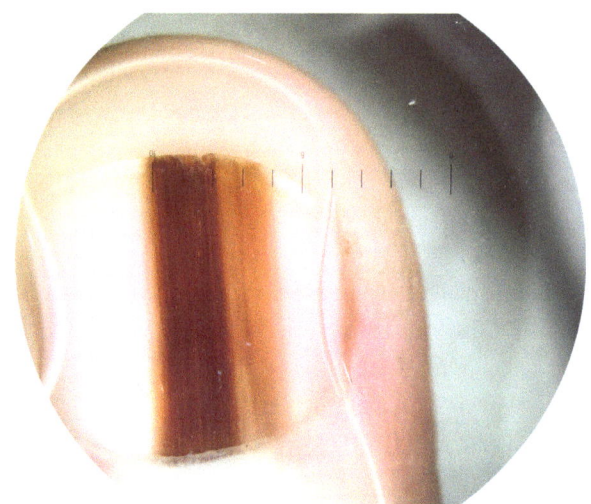

The dermoscopic examination of subungual pigmented lesions is often difficult to interpret and should be done scrupulously. In this case the benign features (like e.g. parallelism of pigmented strias and lack of Hutchinson's sign) were present with malignant ones (like e.g. polychromatosis, dystrophy of the nail plate and a shape of the lesion). Considering anamnesis, clinical and dermoscopic manifestation, the suspicion of subungual melanoma was in the first place.

Subsequently, the excisional biopsy and the histopathological examination of the pigmented lesion of the nail matrix were performed (Figs. 16.3, 16.4, 16.5, and 16.6). Haematoxylin and eosin stain revealed intraepidermal nests of malignant cells (Fig. 16.7), which showed positive reaction for S100 antigen and negative reactivity with cytokeratin 7 (CK 7), cytokeratin 20 (CK 20) and cytokeratin of heavy molecular weight (CK HMW).

Fig. 16.3 Incision of the nail fold

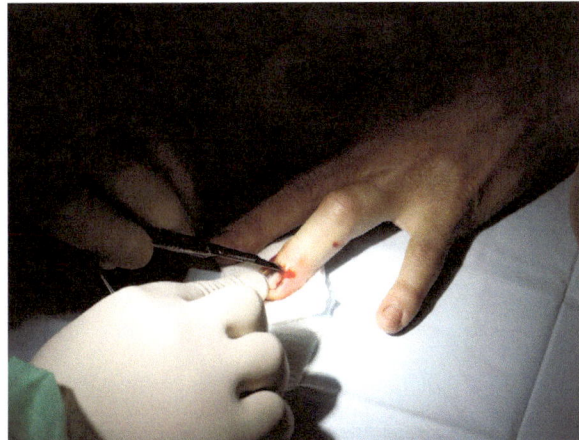

Fig. 16.4 Status after nail plate removal

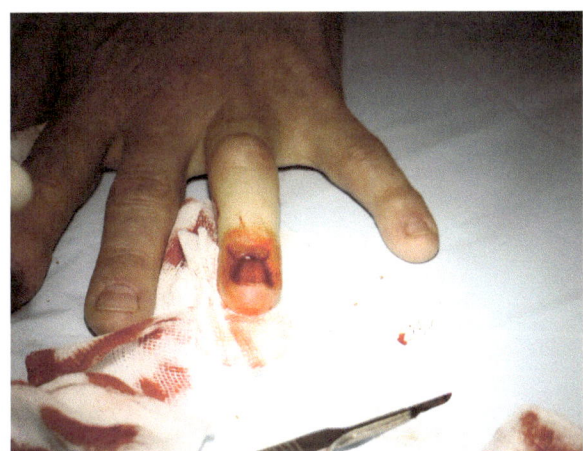

Fig. 16.5 Excisional biopsy of the pigmented lesion of the nail matrix

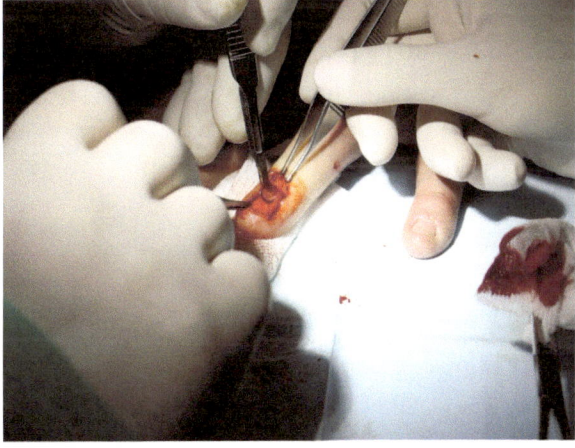

Fig. 16.6 Stitching of the nail fold

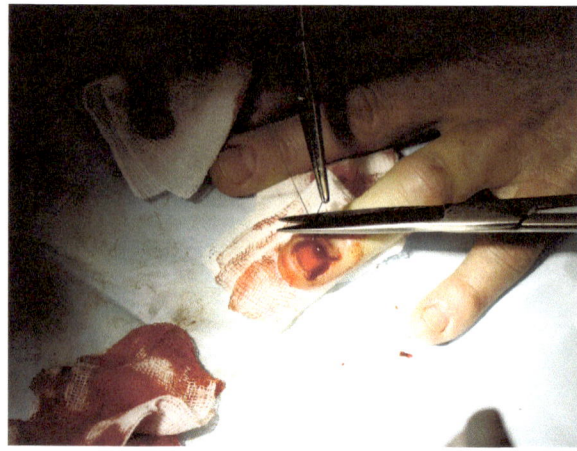

Fig. 16.7 Histology of the subungual pigmented lesion. Diagnosis: Malignant melanoma in situ (haematoxylin & eosin, original magnification x10)

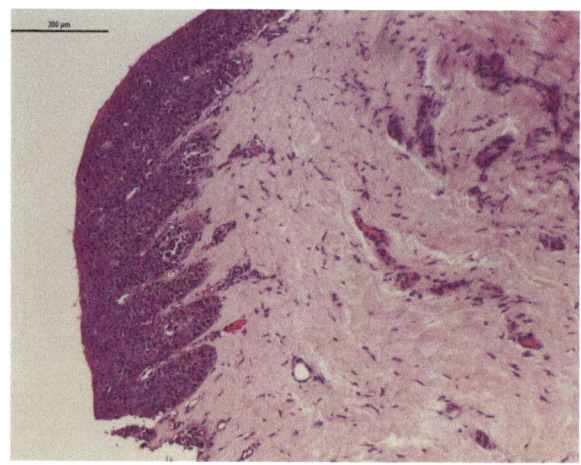

Diagnosis Acral Lentiginous Melanoma (ALM) in situ

Discussion

Melanonychia is characterized by brown to black pigmentation of the normal nail plate, and most often occurs for benign etiologies. It results from increased melanin pigmentation of the nail matrix epithelium and as a result also the nail plate, due to nail matrix melanocytic activation or nail matrix melanocytic hyperplasia, and, sporadically, due to nail invasion by melanin-producing pathogens [1, 2].

Furthermore, brown to black nail pigmentation can also be of non-melanin origin and then, it is usually caused by bacterial or fungal nail infections, exogenous substances, or subungual haemorrhage.

Longitudinal melanonychia most frequently appears as pigmented band due to nail matrix lesion. It may be a sign of many benign lesions, such as subungual melanocytic nevus or lentigo, but may also be the presenting sign of melanoma of the nail unit. Despite the subungual melanoma is infrequent diagnosis, any longitudinal brown band within a single nail plate must be examined and investigated with caution.

During dermatoscopic examination of longitudinal melanonychias the following features should arouse suspicion of subungual melanoma:

- irregular brown pigmentation (variation in colour, blurring),
- grey or black in addition to brown colour,
- granular pigmentation,
- new pigment, especially, if there is no preceding trauma or other explanation,
- width of the lesion over 3 mm or involvement of more than a half of the nail plate,
- Hutchinson's or micro-Hutchinson's sign,
- nail plate dystrophy,
- recurrent spontaneous haemorrhage in the same place,
- distal narrowing of the pigmented bands forming a triangular or trapezoidal shape of the lesion [3, 4].

Although acral lentiginous melanoma (ALM) accounts only for about 2–3% of all melanomas, it definitely comprises greater part of total melanomas in darker-skinned individuals, with blacks having the highest percentage.

This subtype of melanoma is associated with a worse survival rates, than cutaneous malignant melanoma overall. One of the reason for poor prognosis may have been a late diagnosis. Therefore, it is important to examine closely patient's palms, soles, and nail beds, especially regarding blacks, Asians and Hispanics [1].

Careful anamnesis, physical examination and dermoscopy of the nail unit contribute to the proper diagnosis; however, histologic examination still remains the gold standard diagnostic method. Early-stage melanomas can often be cured with surgery. More advanced melanomas might be much difficult to treat. However, in recent years, newer types of immunotherapy and targeted therapies have shown a great promise and have changed the prognosis in the most advanced disease stages [1, 5, 6].

Key Points
- Despite malignant melanoma accounts for less than 2% of all cutaneous malignancies, it still has one of the worst prognosis among patients with these neoplasms.
- Acral lentiginous melanoma, including subungual melanoma, is one of the histologic subtypes of malignant melanoma of bad prognosis.
- Dermoscopy of subungual pigmented lesions is very difficult and should be accomplished thoroughly.

References

1. Rutkowski P, Wysocki PJ, Nasierowska-Guttmejer A, et al. Cutaneous melanomas. Oncol Clin Pract. 2017;13:241–58.
2. Di Chiacchio N, Noriega LF. Melanonychias. In: Tosti A, editor. Nail disorders, vol. 2019: Elsevier. p. 85–95.
3. Kamińska-Winciorek G, Śpiewak R. Dermoscopy on subungual melanoma. Post High Med Dosw. 2013;67:380–7.
4. Tosti A, Piraccini BM, de Farias DC. Dealing with melanonychia. Semin Cutan Med Surg. 2009;28:49–54.
5. Jellinek N. Nail matrix biopsy of longitudinal melanonychia: diagnostic algorithm including the matrix shave biopsy. J Am Acad Dermatol. 2007;56:803–10.
6. Koga H, Saida T, Uhara H. Key point in dermoscopic differentiation between early nail apparatus melanoma and benign longitudinal melanonychia. J Dermatol. 2011;38:45–52.

Chapter 17
A Residual Pigmentary Lesion After Melanoma Surgery

M. Rovesti, C. Feliciani, A. Zucchi, T. Lotti, and F. Satolli

A 90-years-old patient underwent a surgery for a nodule on the vertex with the outcome of non-ulcered nodular melanoma, which was dermis-infiltrating with 2.9 mm Breslow. Associated to the nodular component there was an extended pigmented lesion, as in the Picture 17.1.

A dermoscopy of the residual lesion was made (some details in the Picture 17.2). Based on the case description and the photographs, what is your diagnosis?

1. Ink-spot lentigo
2. Lentigo Maligna
3. Invasive Melanoma
4. Pigmented actinic keratosis

Dermoscopy (showing thick pigmented lines around appendageal openings called rhomboidal structures, asymmetric pigmentation with angulate brown, gray lines and gray dots, dark blotches and obliterated hair follicles) and a biopsy of the residual lesion confirmed the diagnosis of lentigo maligna-melanoma in situ.

Considering the lesion extent, the histological variant (lentigo maligna sort) and the patient's age, it has been decided to treat it with 5% lmiquimod 5 times per weeks for 7 months (with almost complete resolution of the melanoma in situ, see the Picture 17.3) and subsequently with 3.75% Imiquimod for other 2 months, with complete resolution of the Melanoma In Situ.

M. Rovesti (✉) · C. Feliciani · A. Zucchi · F. Satolli
Department of Dermatology, University of Parma, Parma, Italy
e-mail: claudio.feliciani@unipr.it; alfredo.zucchi@unipr.it

T. Lotti
Department of Dermatology and Venereology, University of Rome "G. Marconi" Via Vittoria Colonna, Rome, Italy

Picture 17.1 Residual
pigmentary lesion
after surgery

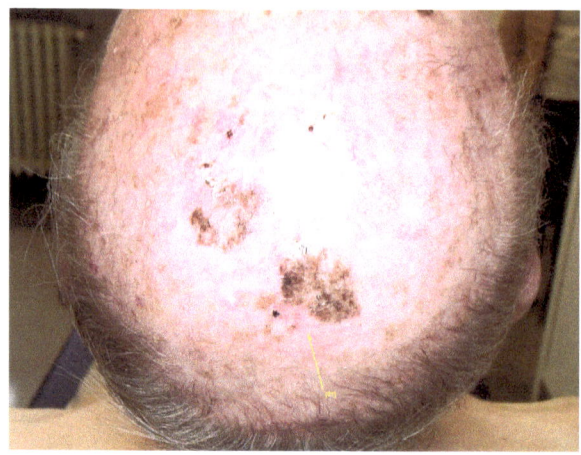

Picture 17.2 Some
dermoscopical features of
the residual
pigmentary lesion

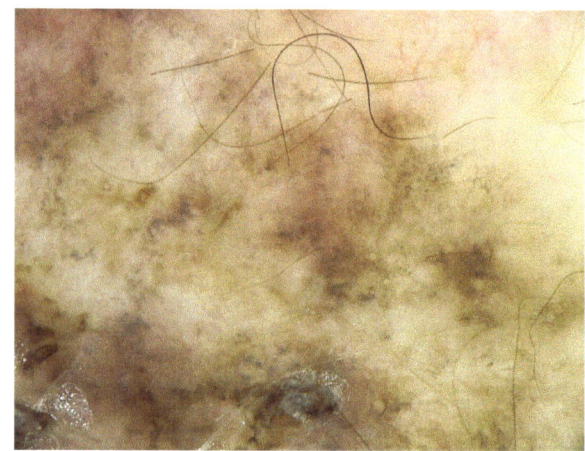

Picture 17.3 Almost
complete resolution of the
lentigo maligna after
7 months of 5% imiquimod

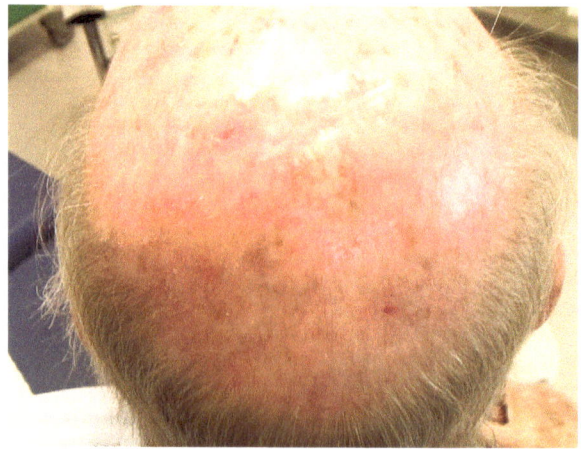

Diagnosis

Lentigo Maligna Melanoma.

Discussion

Lentigo maligna (LM) is an in situ variant of melanoma. Which presents as a slowly enlarging brown to grey black pigmented and sometimes amelanotic macule on chronically sun-exposed skin. In particular, in patient older than 45 years the incidence of LM and LM Melanoma (LMM) is increasing [1].

For the diagnosis and management of LM and LMM dermoscopy is an indispensable tool as suggested by literature [2]; in fact, dermoscopy aided not only the diagnosis (helping the most appropriate area to biopsy, to evaluate the margins of the tumour,…) but allows a non-invasive follow up of treatments, in particular for the topical ones, estimating the assessment of lack of criteria suggestive for tumour persistence. In our patient, a dermoscopy evaluation every two months allowed to continue the topical therapy until the complete response.

About treatments, in international guidelines, recommendations based on expert option state that surgical excision with at least a 5-mm margin is the therapy of first choice [3]. For various reasons, surgical management of LM can be challenging: in case of large lesion, reconstructive procedures may be needed after excision and most patients with LM are elderly and may be frail and suffer from comorbidity, as in our patient.

Over the past 15 years, imiquimod cream has gained attention as an off-label, topical and non-invasive treatment modality for LM.

Topical Imiquimod is a synthetic imidazoquinoline amine with toll-like receptor 7 agonist properties, able to increase the production of inflammatory cytokine and chemokines. Imiquimod also exerts its effect on tumour cell apoptosis through activation of the caspase pathway and has angiogenic effects through the downregulation of fibroblast growth factor and upregulation of inhibitors of angiogenesis.

According to the literature, 5%imiquimod is effective in the treatment of external condylomata acuminata, cutaneous warts, superficial basal cell carcinoma and actinic keratosis [4]. However, recent studies have demonstrated similar efficacy and reported lower complications using 3.75% imiquimod for the treatment of actinic keratosis [5, 6].

Regarding melanoma in situ, we like to underline that imiquimod is currently not approved in the treatment of LM and LMM, however more and more papers support its effectiveness for the treatment of lentigo maligna, as single treatment or after surgery and cryotherapy [7].

Unfortunately, a standard treatment schedule doesn't exist. A systematic review on the role of imiquimod in lentigo maligna and lentigo maligna melanoma [1] concludes that 6–7 applications of 5%imiquimod per week, with at least 60 applications, shows the greatest odds of complete clinical and histological clearance of LM.

In our patient we decided to prefer 5times for week of applications of 5% and then 3.75%imiquimod to reduce the side effects of the treatment and use it for more time (approximately 180 sessions) until complete resolution of the lesion.

In conclusion, topical 5% and 3.75%imiquimod is an option for lentigo maligna in patients unfit for or not willing to undergo surgery or radiotherapy.

Key Points

- Lentigo maligna is an in situ variant of melanoma
- For a correct diagnosis and management of LM and LMM, dermoscopy is an indispensable tool
- Imiquimod is an option for lentigo maligna in patients unfit for or not willing to undergo surgery or radiotherapy.

References

1. Tio D, Van der Woude J, Prinsens CAC, et al. A systematic review on the role of imiquimod in lentigo maligna and lentigo maligna melanoma: need for standardization treatment of treatment schedule and outcome measures. J Eur Acad Dermatol Venereol. 2017;31(4):616–24.
2. Hamilko de Barros M, Conforti C, Giuffrida R, et al. Clinical usefulness of dermoscopy in the management of lentigo maligna melanoma treated with topical imiquimod: a case report. Dermatol Ther. 2019;32:e13048.
3. Garbe C, Peris K, Hauschild A, et al. Diagnosis and treatment of melanoma: European consensus-based interdisciplinary guideline. Eur J Cancer. 2010;46:270–83.
4. Tsay C, Kim S, Norwich-Cavanaugh A, et al. An algorithm for the management of residual head and neck melanoma in situ using topical imiquimod. Ann Plast Surg. 2019;82:S199–201.
5. Swanson N, Abramovits W, Berman B, Kulp J, Rigel DS, Levy S. Imiqui-mod 2.5% and 3.75% for the treatment of actinic keratoses: results of two placebo-controlled studies of daily application to the face and balding scalp for two 2-week cycles. J Am Acad Dermatol. 2010;62:582–90.
6. Swanson N, Smith CC, Kaur M, et al. Imiquimod 2.5% and 3.75% for the treatment of actinic keratoses: two phase 3, multicenter, randomized, double-blind, placebo-controlled studies. J Drugs Dermatol. 2014;13:166–9.
7. Tio D, Van Montfrans C, Ruijter CGH, Hoekzema R, Bekkenk MW. Effectiveness of 5%. Topical imiquimod for lentigo maligna treatment. Acta Derm Venereol. 2019;99:884–8.

Chapter 18
A 45-Year-Old Woman with a Brown Spot on the Right Arm

Monica Popescu, Carmen Maria Salavastru, and George-Sorin Tiplica

A 45-year-old female attended the Dermatology Clinic in 2014 for a pigmentary tumor on the antero-lateral aspect of the right arm. She noticed the change of a pre-existing "brown spot" for the last two years (Clinical images: Fig. 18.1 and dermoscopy: Fig. 18.2). During the last 12 months, the patient noticed the apparition of the dark and blue pigmentations, of a small nodule and the increase in size of the tumor.

Her medical history revealed an invasive ductal carcinoma breast cancer type G3 that was diagnosed in 2008. The immunohistochemistry result showed: Estrogen receptors (ER) alpha DAKO clone 1D5 positive 20% intensity +, Progesterone receptors (PR) DAKO clone PgR 636 positive 60% intensity +, C-erbB2/HER2 oncoprotein = 2 +, Ki-67 DAKO nuclear antigen clones MIB-1 = 3% and Cytokeratin 5/6 DAKO clone D5/16 B4 cytoplasmic = negative. She underwent left mastectomy with lymphadenectomy of intra-pectoral ganglion groups and chemotherapy with Epirubicin Hydrochloride (180 mg) and Cyclophosphamide (1200 mg/2 mp). She received tamoxifen hormone therapy during 2008–2010. The patient is also known to have high-risk stage I arterial hypertension.

Based on the case description and the clinical and dermoscopy photographs, what is your diagnosis?

M. Popescu
Dermatology Research Unit, Colentina Clinical Hospital, Bucharest, Romania

Carol Davila University of Medicine and Pharmacy, Bucharest, Romania

C. M. Salavastru (✉)
Carol Davila University of Medicine and Pharmacy, Bucharest, Romania

Pediatric Dermatology Department, Colentina Clinical Hospital, Bucharest, Romania

G.-S. Tiplica
Carol Davila University of Medicine and Pharmacy, Bucharest, Romania

Second Dermatology Clinic, Colentina Clinical Hospital, Bucharest, Romania

T. Lotti et al. (eds.), *Clinical Cases in Melanoma*,
Clinical Cases in Dermatology, https://doi.org/10.1007/978-3-030-50820-3_18

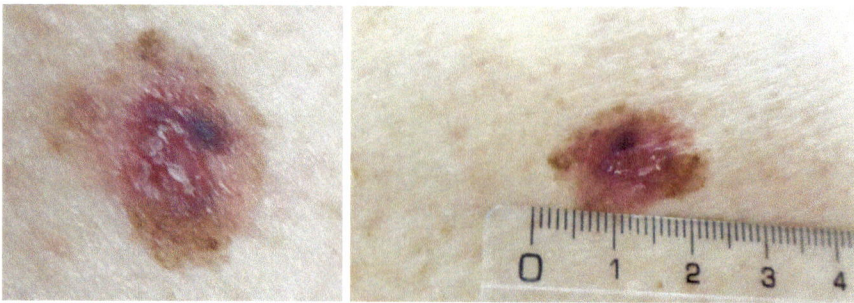

Fig. 18.1 Asymmetric pigmentary tumor on the antero-lateral aspect of the right arm, ill-defined, with multiple colours (various shades of pink, grey-blue and brown) and a diameter of 2 cm

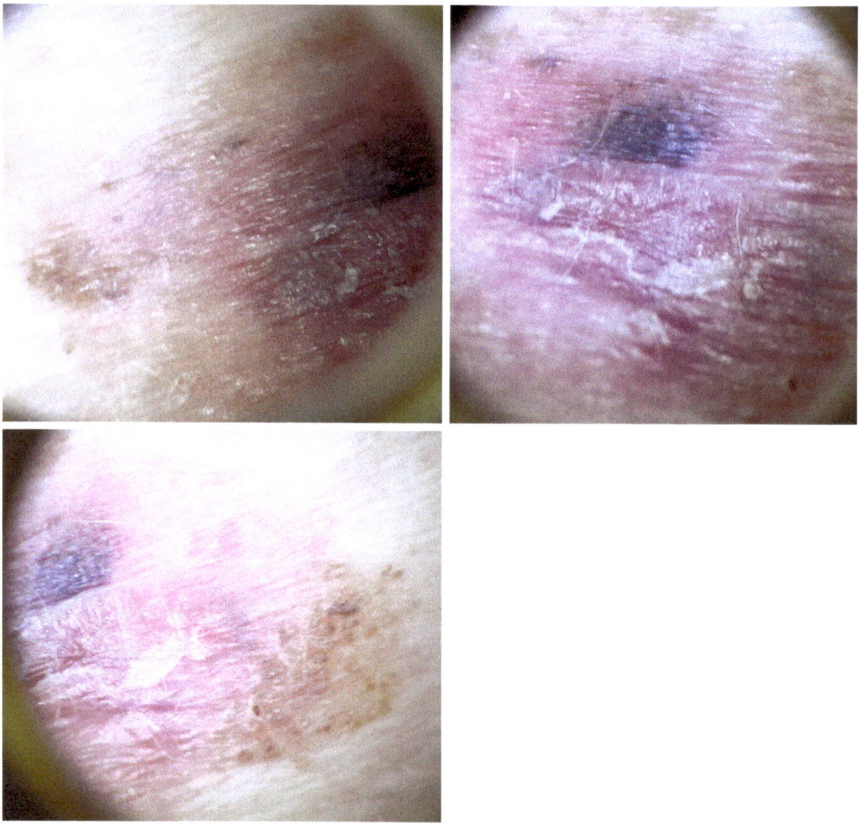

Fig. 18.2 Dermoscopy images: Asymmetric and ill-defined tumor with atypical pigment network, peripheric globules, abrupt border, grey-blue structure and pink structureless area

1. Cutaneous metastasis of the brest carcinoma
2. Bowen's disease
3. Pigmented basal cell carcinoma
4. Superficial Spreading Melanoma
5. Dermatofibrosarcoma protuberans

Surgical excision with one centimeter margins was performed. The histology confirmed the diagnosis of Superficial Spreading Melanoma with invasive vertical growth, developed on a melanocytic nevus (Figs. 18.3 and 18.4). The Breslow thickness was 1.1 mm with positive perivascular invasion and 4 mitosis/mm^2 mitotic rate. There was no ulceration, perineural invasion, tumor regression or satellite nodules found. The stage of the tumour was pT$_{2a}$pNxMx (according to AJCC 7th edition).

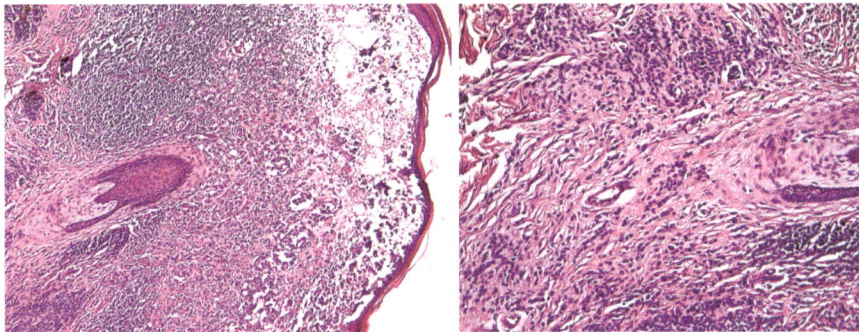

Fig. 18.3 Superficial Spreading Melanoma with invasive vertical growth, developed on a melanocytic nevus with atypical melanocytes arranged singly or in clusters in the epidermis

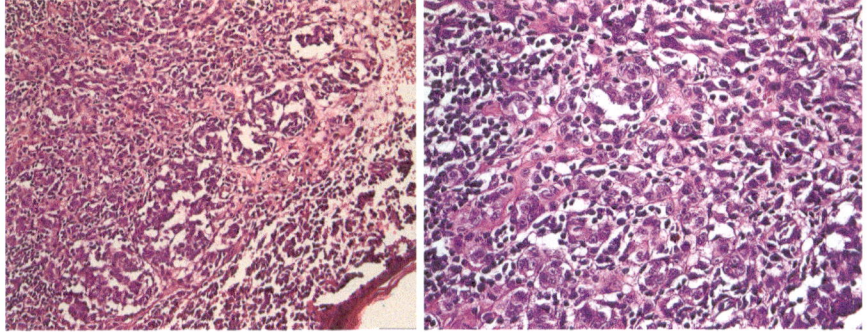

Fig. 18.4 The tumor cells are epithelioid with abundant cytoplasm, pleomorphic nuclei, prominent nucleoli, organised in nests and clusters

Diagnosis

Superficial Spreading Melanoma (SSM) stage IB (AJCC seventh edition) developed on melanocytic nevus in a patient with history of invasive ductal carcinoma breast cancer (BC).

Discussion

Given their prognostic implications, cutaneous metastases represent an important dermatologic entity. Cutaneous metastases develop an average of 36 months (range, 1 to 177 months) after the initial diagnosis of the primary malignancy. In women, BC and melanoma are the malignancies that most frequently metastasize to the skin. When a patient with a known history of cancer presents with an extremely rapidly growing nodule or an eruption of multiple skin nodules in close proximity to the primary tumor, the diagnosis of cutaneous metastasis is relatively straightforward. However, the skin lesions may grow more slowly, and while metastases typically appear within several years of the diagnosis of the primary malignancy, they can present decades later. Of all the carcinomas that metastasize to the skin, BC may be the one with the widest range of clinical lesions, varying from papulonodules to patches of erythema mimicking erysipelas (inflammatory carcinoma) to woody induration.

Rarely, epidermotropic metastases, especially from breast carcinoma, may contain pigment and even an intratumoral increase in melanocytes, leading to the misdiagnosis of a melanocytic tumor [1].

Squamous cell carcinoma (SCC) *in situ*, commonly called Bowen's disease, is a keratinocyte carcinoma. The most common presentation of SCC *in situ* is an erythematous scaly patch or slightly elevated plaque that often arises within sun-exposed skin of an elderly individual. The head and neck, followed by the extremities and trunk, are the most common sites [1]. The most typical dermoscopic features of Bowen's disease include glomerular vessels and scaly surface. Although dermoscopy of Bowen's disease has been well established other skin lesions may present similar or identical structures in dermoscopic images leading to differential diagnosis dilemmas. Histopathological confirmation should be obtained prior the treatment of suspected cases of Bowen's disease in order to avoid a misdiagnosis [2].

Basal cell carcinoma (BCC) is a keratinocyte carcinoma and represents the most frequently observed malignancy among Caucasians. Pigmented BCCs usually have the overall architecture of a nodular BCC. They contain aggregates of melanin, often irregularly distributed and melanocytes [1]. Dermoscopy of pigmented BCC presents pigment globules, maple leaf structures, and one arborizing telangiectasia as well as a pink background color [1].

SSM is the most common type of cutaneous melanoma in fair-skinned individuals and it is diagnosed most frequently between the ages of 40 and 60 years. About half of SSMs arise in a pre-existing nevus though the likelihood of an individual nevus progressing to melanoma is exceedingly low [1].

Skin produces sex hormones as neuromediators for homeostasis. An interesting development in estrogen receptor research is the second type of estrogen receptor, estrogen receptor beta (ERb). Most of the research on both ERa and ERb has been in the area of breast cancer research, where the former is important in determining response to endocrine therapy. As for dermatologic implications, Schmidt et al. investigated specific immunostaining patterns of both ERa and ERb in benign nevi, dysplastic nevi with "mild, moderate, and severe" cytologic atypia, lentigo malignas, and melanomas. ERb was the predominant receptor type found in all of the melanocytic lesions studied. A strong correlation was seen with ERb expression and the proximity of melanoma cells to keratinocytes, that is, expression was most intense in melanoma cells in the epidermis and in the papillary dermis close to the epidermis, compared with melanoma cells deeper in the dermis [3].

An equally important type of ER is the G protein-coupled estrogen receptor (GPER). GPER belongs to G protein-coupled receptor family of cellular membrane molecules that are found to be involved in development and progression of different cancer types. In skin, it regulates melanin production and is expressed in melanoma cells. It promotes melanogenesis via an intracellular pathway resulting in increasing cAMP levels. There is a subsequent activation of intracellular cAMP-protein kinase to an elevation of CREB phosphorylation as well as activation of microphthalmia-associated transcription factor (MITF). This latter regulates melanocyte growth, differentiation and function [4].

Tamoxifen is a nonsteroidal triphenylethylene derivative that binds to the estrogen receptor. It remains the standard therapy for women with estrogen receptor-positive breast carcinoma. It has both estrogenic and antiestrogenic actions, depending on the target tissue. Tamoxifen inhibits melanoma cell proliferation invasion and metastasis, but the targets of tamoxifen in melanoma remain unclear. The actions of tamoxifen are generally believed to involve the actions of estrogen receptors such as GPER. Tamoxifen individually has provided extremely poor response rates (less than 10%) in melanoma clinical trials [5].

Oestrogen dependency is attributed to a number of cancers, including breast cancer; however, there is still growing evidence that melanoma should also be cited as a hormonally dependent tumour. This comes from the observations of gender-related differences in melanoma progression and reports concerning the history of the malignant course of melanomas during pregnancy. Observations of the influence of oestrogen on melanoma cells are controversial despite the fact that there is a great deal of contradiction in the results concerning the role of oestrogen in the course of melanomas. On one hand, there is still growing clinical and preclinical evidence suggesting that oestrogen stimulation does have an influence on melanoma cells and may regulate their metastatic progression [6]. On the other hand, some studies described a lower melanoma risk for women treated with antiestrogens, such as tamoxifen, which can also be used in the treatment of stage IV melanoma.

MDA-MB-435 Breast and UCLA-SO-M14 Melanoma cell lines share a common origin. The authenticity of two cell lines, has been debated in the scientific literature over many years. Questions were first raised regarding the tissue origin of MDA-MB-435 in 2000, when cDNA microarray analysis of the NCI-60 panel showed that the expression pattern of the claimed breast carcinoma cells closely resembled patterns seen in melanoma cell lines. Subsequent analysis of multiple samples of MDA-MB-435 showed that cell stocks in use at different laboratories around the world shared common expression patterns associated with melanoma. Numerous analytical approaches (karyotyping, comparative genomic hybridization, microsatellite polymorphism analysis, STR analysis, single nucleotide polymorphism analysis and bioinformatics analysis of gene expression) have demonstrated the common origin of the melanoma and breast cancer cell line [7]. Studies showed that patients with breast cancer might have a greater risk of developing melanoma, especially if they are carriers of the breast cancer susceptibility gene BRCA2. Also, epidemiological data documented that the connection can be bi-directional, with women diagnosed with primary melanoma later developing breast carcinoma [8].

Melanoma arising on the arm is not a frequent locations for melanoma (the arm is not associated with maximal sun exposure). In our case, the two year period of Tamoxifen therapy and the location of melanoma may suggest a stronger risk factors for induction the melanoma than UV exposure and the sensitivity of melanocytes to estrogens.

As for clinical and laboratory evidence concerning hormones, nevi, and melanoma, a clear link has not been demonstrated between endogenous (pregnancy) and exogenous (hormone replacement therapy) hormones and melanoma. The demonstration of ERb receptors in dysplastic nevi and certain melanoma is interesting, but further research is needed in this area to determine the relevance of this observation [3]. Dermatofibrosarcoma protuberans (DFSP) is a soft tissue malignancy characterized by slow, locally invasive growth. Typically arising in the dermis of the skin, DFSP is usually found on the torso and less commonly on the arms, legs, and neck [9]. DFSP has a low rate of metastatic spread, however, its local growth can be destructive and disfiguring if left untreated or if treatment is delayed. On clinical examination, DFSP commonly appears as a salmon-colored erythematous plaque, extending into the subcutaneous tissue, fascia, and adjacent muscle with tendril-like growth and microscopic extensions, which can make complete surgical resection difficult [10].

Based on the clinical, dermoscopic images and histology result, the diagnosis of SSM developed on a melanocytic nevus of the antero-lateral face of the right arm with a 1.1 mm Breslow was made. The patient underwent excision with 1 cm margins (complete resection) and, subsequentelly, sentinel lymph node biopsy, followed by lymphadenectomy of 12 right axillary lymph nodes. The histology showed that the lymph nodes were not invaded.

The patient was instructed to avoid sun exposure and regular clinical follow-up including review of systems, full skin examination and oncologic evaluation every 3–12 months for 5 years and then annually as clinically indicated.

Key Points

- About half of SSMs arise in a pre-existing nevus although the likelihood of an individual nevus progressing to melanoma is exceedingly low.
- MDA-MB-435 Breast and UCLA-SO-M14 Melanoma cell lines share a common origin.
- There was found evidence for a bidirectional association between breast cancer and cutaneous melanoma.
- Tamoxifen has both estrogenic and antiestrogenic actions. Observations of the influence of oestrogen on melanoma cells are controversial.
- Our case may suggest a stronger risk factors for induction the melanoma than UV exposure and the sensitivity of melanocytes to estrogens.

References

1. Bolognia JL, Schaffer JV, Cerroni L. Dermatology. 4th ed. London: Elsevier; 2017.
2. Wozniak-Rito AM, Rudnicka L. Bowen's disease in dermoscopy. Acta Dermatovenerol Croat. 2018 Jun;26(2):157–61.
3. Marcia S Driscoll, Jane M Grant-Kels. Hormones, nevi, and melanoma: an approach to the patient. JAAD December 2007;57, number 6.
4. Dika E, Annalisa P, Lambertini M, Manuelpillai N, Fiorentino M, Altimari A, Ferracin M, Mattia L, Fabbri E, Campione E, Veronesi G, Scarfi F. Estrogen receptors and melanoma: a review. Cells. 2019; Published: 19 November 2019.
5. Ribeiro MPC, Santos AE, Custódio JBA. Rethinking tamoxifen in the management of melanoma: new answers for an old question. Eur J Pharmacol. 2015;764:372–8.
6. Janik ME, Bełkot K, Przybyło M. Is oestrogen an important player in melanoma progression? Contemp Oncol (Pozn). 2014;18(5):302–6.
7. Korch C, Hall EM, Dirks WG, Ewing M, Faries M, Varella-Garcia M, Robinson S, Storts D, Turner JA, Wang Y, Burnett EC, Healy L, Kniss D, Neve RM, Nims RW, Reid YA, Robinson WA, Capes-Davis A. Authentication of M14 melanoma cell line proves misidentification of MDA-MB-435 breast cancer cell line. Int J Cancer. 2018 Feb 1;142(3):561–72.
8. Wolfe J. The association between melanoma and breast cancer and implications for care. Cutaneous Oncol Today. 2011;Oct:10–13.
9. McArthur G. Dermatofibrosarcoma protuberans: recent clinical progress. Ann Surg Oncol. 2007;14(10):2876–86.
10. Johnson-Jahangir H, Sherman W, Ratner D. Using imatinib as neoadjuvant therapy in dermatofibrosarcoma protuberans: potential pluses and minuses. J Natl Compr Cancer Netw. 2010;8(8):881–5.

Chapter 19
A Deep Nodule of the Left Arm in a 49-Year-Old Woman

Stefana Cretu, Carmen Maria Salavastru, and George-Sorin Tiplica

We present the case of a 49-year old Caucasian female patient, diagnosed in April 2012 with metastatic melanoma with unknown primary (MUP). This diagnosis was made by the excision of an intradermal nodul situated on her left arm, when histopathological examination established the diagnosis of melanoma metastasis. No primary tumour could be identified. The patient also had involvement of the lymph nodes and bone (left femur) (TxN1M1). The tumour tested positive for BRAF (V600E) mutation and the patient started therapy with vemurafenib.

Before the onset of vemurafenib therapy, in October 2012, a complete dermatological examination was performed and more than 100 melanocytic nevi were identified. Some of the lesions were removed, with the pathology report concluding they were benign.

Five months after initiation of BRAF inhibitor therapy, in February 2013, after missing three monthly follow-up visits, the patient presented for her dermatological screening. It was noticed, by dermatoscopy, a worrisome aspect of a melanocytic lesion located on the right medial axillary line (Fig. 19.1).

Also, on the same visit, the patient presented with multiple wide-spred hyperkeratotic papules affecting the trunk; a punch-biopsy was performed.

S. Cretu
Dermatology Research Unit, Colentina Clinical Hospital, Bucharest, Romania

Carol Davila University of Medicine and Pharmacy, Bucharest, Romania

C. M. Salavastru (✉)
Carol Davila University of Medicine and Pharmacy, Bucharest, Romania

Pediatric Dermatology Department, Colentina Clinical Hospital, Bucharest, Romania

G.-S. Tiplica
Carol Davila University of Medicine and Pharmacy, Bucharest, Romania

Second Dermatology Clinic, Colentina Clinical Hospital, Bucharest, Romania

© The Editor(s) (if applicable) and The Author(s), under exclusive license to
Springer Nature Switzerland AG 2020
T. Lotti et al. (eds.), *Clinical Cases in Melanoma*,
Clinical Cases in Dermatology, https://doi.org/10.1007/978-3-030-50820-3_19

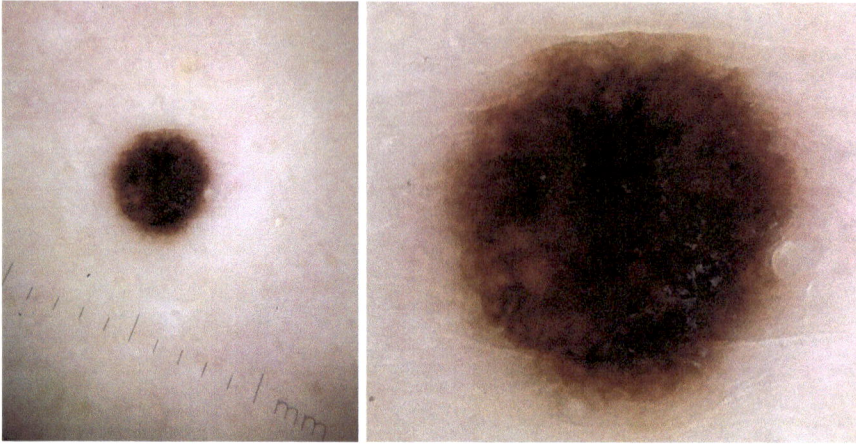

Fig. 19.1 Dermatoscopic examination of the melanoma located on the right medial axillary line and hyperkeratosis

Eight months after the onset of Vemurafenib treatment the patient presented with an ulcerated nodular non melanocytic tumour located on her right calf. The lesion was surgically removed.

Based on the case description and the photographs, what is your diagnosis?

Atypical melanocytic lesion located on the trunk:

1. Melanoma
2. Melanoma metastasis
3. Atypical nevus

Hyperkeratotic eruption:

1. Drug induced rash (acantholytic diskeratosis Darier-like)
2. Darier's disease
3. Grover's disease

Non-melanocytic tumor on the right calf:

1. Amelanotic melanoma
2. Basal cell carcinoma
3. Squamous cell carcinoma
4. Melanoma metastasis

The histopathology examination and immunohistochemistry of the pigmentary lesion revealed a superficial spreading melanoma in situ with Breslow's depth 0.35 mm. No mitotic activity, ulceration, regression or invasion were observed (Fig. 19.2) (pTis pNx).

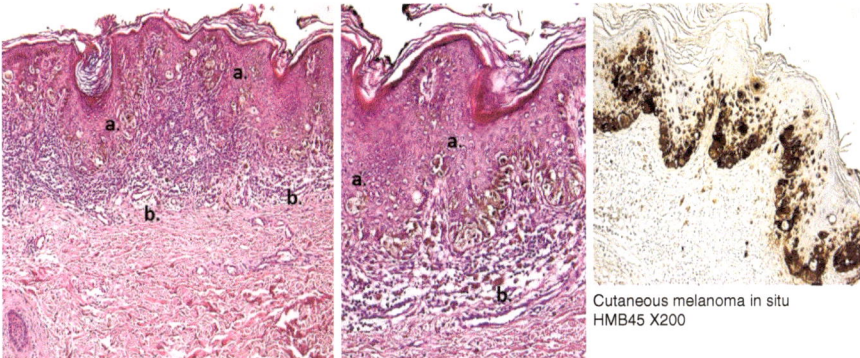

Cutaneous melanoma in situ HE X100 and x200

a. Increased number of melanocytes with atypical nuclei in single cells and small nests located at
   the dermo-epidermal junction and at all levels of the epidermis (Pagetoid spread)
b. Marked presence of inflammatory infiltrate in the dermis, with high number of melanophages

Fig. 19.2 Histopathologic and immunohistochemistry images of the melanoma located on the right medial axillary line

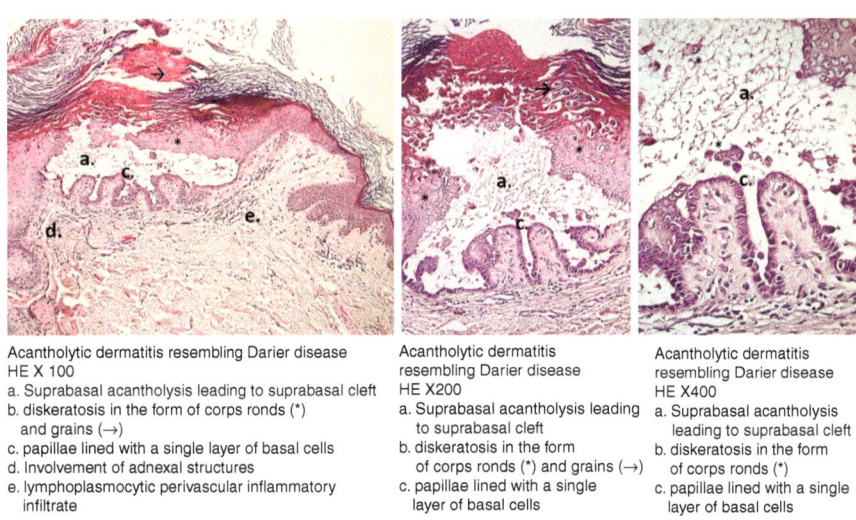

Acantholytic dermatitis resembling Darier disease
HE X 100
a. Suprabasal acantholysis leading to suprabasal cleft
b. diskeratosis in the form of corps ronds (*)
   and grains (→)
c. papillae lined with a single layer of basal cells
d. Involvement of adnexal structures
e. lymphoplasmocytic perivascular inflammatory
   infiltrate

Acantholytic dermatitis
resembling Darier disease
HE X200
a. Suprabasal acantholysis leading
   to suprabasal cleft
b. diskeratosis in the form
   of corps ronds (*) and grains (→)
c. papillae lined with a single
   layer of basal cells

Acantholytic dermatitis
resembling Darier disease
HE X400
a. Suprabasal acantholysis
   leading to suprabasal cleft
b. diskeratosis in the form
   of corps ronds (*)
c. papillae lined with a single
   layer of basal cells

Fig. 19.3 Histopathologic image of acantholytic dyskeratosis resembling Darier's disease

The histopathological examination of the punch biopsy taken from one of the hyperkeratotic papules, situated on the posterior thorax revealed intraepidermal acantholysis, mostly suprabasal, with aspect suggesting Darier's disease (Fig. 19.3).

For the nodular ulcerated lesion on the calf the histopathology report indicated a keratoacanthoma-like squamous cell carcinoma, with moderate differentiation, G2 anaplasia grade, tumoral thickness 2.25 mm, pT1Nx (Fig. 19.4).

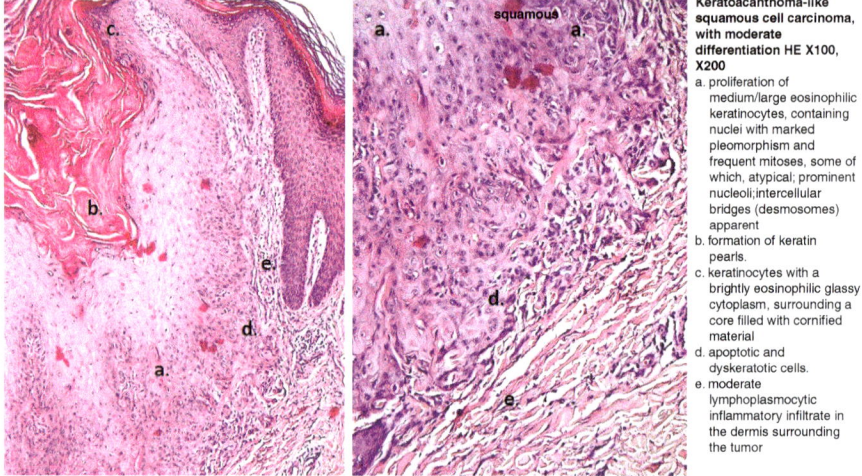

Keratoacanthoma-like squamous cell carcinoma, with moderate differentiation HE X100, X200

a. proliferation of medium/large eosinophilic keratinocytes, containing nuclei with marked pleomorphism and frequent mitoses, some of which, atypical; prominent nucleoli;intercellular bridges (desmosomes) apparent
b. formation of keratin pearls.
c. keratinocytes with a brightly eosinophilic glassy cytoplasm, surrounding a core filled with cornified material
d. apoptotic and dyskeratotic cells.
e. moderate lymphoplasmocytic inflammatory infiltrate in the dermis surrounding the tumor

Fig. 19.4 Histopathologic image of keratoacanthoma-like squamous cell carcinoma, with moderate differentiation (G2 anaplasia grade)

Diagnosis

(a) Second primary melanoma
(b) Acantholytic dyskeratosis resembling Darier's disease
(c) Keratoacanthoma-like quamous cell carcinoma, with moderate differentiation (G2 anaplasia grade)

in a patient with stage IV metastatic melanoma with unknown primary, positive for BRAF (V600E) mutation, receiving tyrosine kinase inhibitors treatment.

Discussion

Tyrosine kinase inhibitors have improved the care of patients suffering from cancer. They have significantly prolonged the survival of patients with advanced melanoma in comparison to former drugs (e.g. dacarbazine). However, as all drugs, they have side-effects and limitations.

BRAF inhibitors (BRAFi) are amongst the first drugs discovered for targeting melanoma mutated cells, through the inhibition of a dysfunctional tyrosine kinase, product of a mutated gene, BRAF^{V600}. Amongst the mutations affecting this gene, BRAF^{V600E} is the one most commonly found in cutaneous melanomas. Because of the mutation, these cells have an increased activity of the mitogen activated protein kinase (MAPK) signalling pathway, resulting in increased proliferation and inhibition of apoptosis [1].

Although effective in growths arrest and limiting the progression of the disease, the BRAFi were also associated with the development of squamous cell carcinomas (SCC) in 12% of cases. This effect seems to be caused by the paradoxical activation of the MAPK pathway in BRAF wildtype cells. The median time to SCC development was 8–12 weeks after onset of vemurafenib therapy [1–3].

In approximately 1% of cases treated with vemurafenib a second primary melanoma developed [1]. This finding may partly be explained by the fact that the MAPK signalling pathway can also be activated by products of mutated genes from other gene families such as MEK1/2, RAS, NF1, PI3K/Akt, PTEN and ERK, a phenomenon known as extrinsic resistance. Within the melanoma tumours several mutated cell lines may coexist, and the inhibition of one line, may lead to the selection of another.

However, even in tumour cell lines having only the BRAF^{V600} mutation, resistance may occur through intrinsic mechanisms, leading to MAPK pathway over activation.

After a median time of 6–8 months, 50% of patients receiving vemurafenimb monotherapy develop melanoma resistance to BRAFi [1–3]. For this reason, new tyrosine kinase inhibitors, such as MEK inhibitors have been associated to BRAFi, with good results regarding patient survival and disease free progression [1–3]. Treatment with BRAFi produces alterations in pre-existing melanocytic lesions and in some cases leads to the development a new primary melanoma within them. This phenomenon may be due to paradoxical activation of BRAF-wildtype in nevus cells by the BRAFi [4]. However, patients diagnosed with one melanoma have an overall higher risk for the development of a second primary lesion even in the absence of BRAFi therapy [5].

In our case, the patient underwent complete dermatologic examination prior to BRAFi therapy initiation, with removal of several melanocytic lesions.

The presence of the drug induced hyperkeratotic maculopapular rash is a common finding during therapy with tyrosine kinase inhibitors that disrupt the MEK and MAPK signalling pathways. This side-effect results from alteration of epidermal homeostasis and the triggering of an acute stress response from the keratinocytes [6].

In patients treated with vemurafenib, Chu et al. identified the presence of acantholytic dyskeratosis in 57% of patients affected, including warty dyskeratoma, Grover or Darier's disease like rashes. The clinical aspect described is similar to that of our patient. In our case the histopathology examination identified all of the features consistent with Darier's disease and involvement of adnexal structures. In the same study, the authors found the presence of keratoacanthoma like squamous cell carcinoma in 29% of patients treated with vemurafenib. Unlike in their cases, where the tumours were well differentiated, our patient had moderate differentiation degree [7].

Key Points

BRAFi have offered great benefits to patients suffering from advanced melanoma. However, adverse drug reactions are to be expected, from which, development of squamous cell carcinomas and second primary melanomas are particularly important and close monitoring should be performed in order to manage these conditions in their earliest phases.

References

1. Kim A, Cohen MS. The discovery of vemurafenib for the treatment of BRAF-mutated metastatic melanoma. Expert Opin Drug Discovery. 2016 Sep 1;11(9):907–16.
2. Mackiewicz J, Mackiewicz A. BRAF and MEK inhibitors in the era of immunotherapy in melanoma patients. Contemp Oncol. 2018 Mar;22(1A):68.
3. Welsh SJ, Rizos H, Scolyer RA, Long GV. Resistance to combination BRAF and MEK inhibition in metastatic melanoma: where to next? Eur J Cancer. 2016 Jul 1;62:76–85.
4. Gerami P, Sorrell J, Martini M. Dermatoscopic evolution of dysplastic nevi showing high-grade dysplasia in a metastatic melanoma patient on vemurafenib. J Am Acad Dermatol. 2012 Dec 1;67(6):e275–6.
5. Debarbieux S, Dalle S, Depaepe L, Poulalhon N, Balme B, Thomas L. Second primary melanomas treated with BRAF blockers: study by reflectance confocal microscopy. Br J Dermatol. 2013 Jun;168(6):1230–5.
6. Schad K, Conzett KB, Zipser MC, Enderlin V, Kamarashev J, French LE, Dummer R. Mitogen-activated protein/extracellular signal-regulated kinase kinase inhibition results in biphasic alteration of epidermal homeostasis with keratinocytic apoptosis and pigmentation disorders. Clin Cancer Res. 2010 Feb 1;16(3):1058–64.
7. Chu EY, Wanat KA, Miller CJ, Amaravadi RK, Fecher LA, Brose MS, McGettigan S, Giles LR, Schuchter LM, Seykora JT, Rosenbach M. Diverse cutaneous side effects associated with BRAF inhibitor therapy: a clinicopathologic study. J Am Acad Dermatol. 2012 Dec 1;67(6):1265–72.

Chapter 20
A Young Woman with a Brown Nail Stripe

Adelina-Maria Sendrea, Carmen Maria Salavastru, and George-Sorin Tiplica

A 36-year old female patient, with no personal or family medical history, presented with longitudinal melanonychia (LM) of the right index, in January 2013. The initial clinical and dermoscopy examination revealed longitudinal homogenous pigmented stria with no width and color variation, without any known local trauma. A nail matrix biopsy was performed and no alterations were found, hence the patient was scheduled for follow-up visits.

The patient was closely monitored, clinically and dermoscopically and in July 2014, a second matrix biopsy was performed, since a slight accentuation of the melanonychia was noticed. No Hutchinson or pseudo-Hutchinson sign were present (Fig. 20.1).

In January 2016, after several follow-up visits, the patient reported a sudden darkening of the pigmented area and the clinical and dermoscopy examination revealed increased pigmentation of stria and onichodistrophy corresponding to the area where the former matrix biopsies were performed with no Hutchinson or pseudo-Hudchinson signs present.

The patient was scheduled for total matrixectomy.

A.-M. Sendrea
Dermatology Research Unit, Colentina Clinical Hospital, Bucharest, Romania

Carol Davila University of Medicine and Pharmacy, Bucharest, Romania

C. M. Salavastru (✉)
Carol Davila University of Medicine and Pharmacy, Bucharest, Romania

Pediatric Dermatology Department, Colentina Clinical Hospital, Bucharest, Romania

G.-S. Tiplica
Carol Davila University of Medicine and Pharmacy, Bucharest, Romania

Second Dermatology Clinic, Colentina Clinical Hospital, Bucharest, Romania

T. Lotti et al. (eds.), *Clinical Cases in Melanoma*,
Clinical Cases in Dermatology, https://doi.org/10.1007/978-3-030-50820-3_20

91

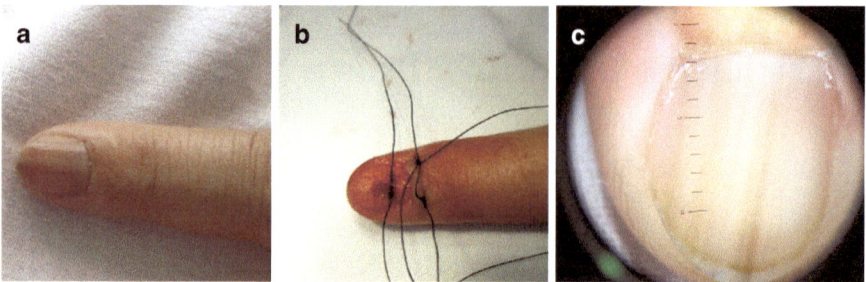

Fig. 20.1 Longitudinal melanonychia of the right index (July 2014): (**a**) clinical, (**b**) post biopsy and (**c**) dermoscopy

Based on your case description and the pictures, what is your diagnosis?

1. Nail unit melanoma
2. Nail matrix nevus
3. Pigmented onychomatricoma
4. Subungual hematoma
5. Blue nevus nail matrix

Taking into account that an adult patient presented with a single digit longitudinal melanonychia, located on the index, a high suspicion of nail unit melanoma seemed reasonable and multiple tests were performed. The initial nail clipping analysis revealed small pigment deposits—possibly melanin (Fontana Masson stain) and no fungal elements (PAS stain) or hemosiderin deposits (Perls stain) and no pathological changes of the nail matrix. Additionally, patient was regularly assessed and at the 18 months follow up, the histopathological evaluation of new samples didn't revealed any pathological changes in the nail clip, nail bed or nail matrix (Fig. 20.2).

In January 2016, after several follow-up visits, as the patient suddenly presented a significant widening of the pigmented band, a total matrixectomy was finally agreed by the patient and therefore, scheduled.

The first histopathological report revealed nevus-like proliferation of cells, located at the dermo-epidermal junction, with lentiginous disposition and a significantly hyperpigmentation of the keratinous component, suggestive for lentigo simplex.

A second histopathological opinion was requested and showed junctional proliferation of melanocytes with both focal lentiginous disposition and nests with tahychromatic, hypertrophic nuclei; additionally, a pagetoid ascension of the tumoral melanocytes in the entire thickness of the pavimentous epithelium and minimally lymphocytic inflammatory infiltrate with frequent melanocytes located subepithelial were identified. Furthermore, the immunohistochemical analysis revealed positive HMB45 and T311, without any dermal component and negative p16, p21 and Ki67. All histopathological findings were consistent with in situ lentiginous melanocytic proliferation with cytonuclear and architectural atipia, enclosing the lesion as part of a spectrum between junctional lentiginous dysplastic melanocytic nevus and in situ acral lentiginous melanoma.

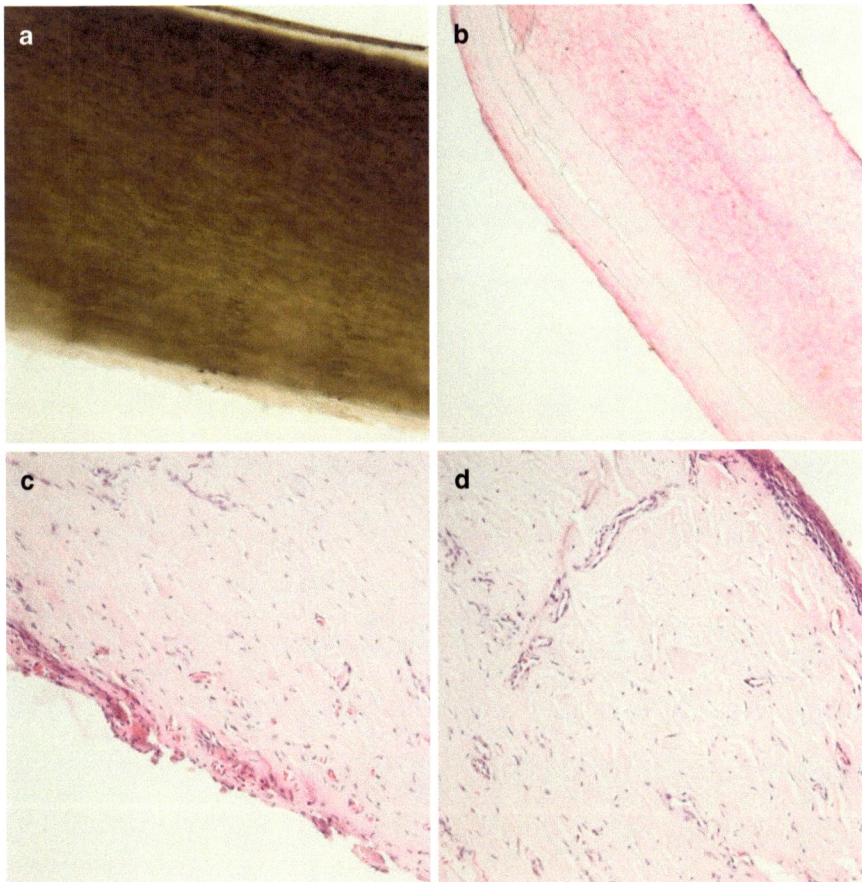

Fig. 20.2 Longitudinal melanonychia of the right index—histopathological aspect (July 2014): (**a**) normal nail plate (Fontana Masson stain 200×); (**b**) normal nail plate (hematoxylin eosin stain 200×); (**c**) normal nail bed (hematoxylin eosin stain 200×); (**d**) normal nail matrix (hematoxylin eosin stain 200×)

A third histopathological reanalysis identified a proliferation of atypical melanocytes located strictly on an epithelial level, with only a vague tendency to nests formation at a junctional and suprajunctional level. The atypical melanocytes presented with small and medium sizes, fusiform, pleomorphic, oval, intensively hyperchromatic nuclei and intensively pigmented cytoplasm and were distributed in an irregular pattern in the matrix, plate, nail folds and hyponychium. Additionally, few melanophages were identified in the underlying dermis. Therefore, the final histopathological diagnosis was of primary in situ non-ulcerated melanoma of the nail apparatus (Fig. 20.3).

Following this diagnosis, a distal phalanx amputation of the right index was performed.

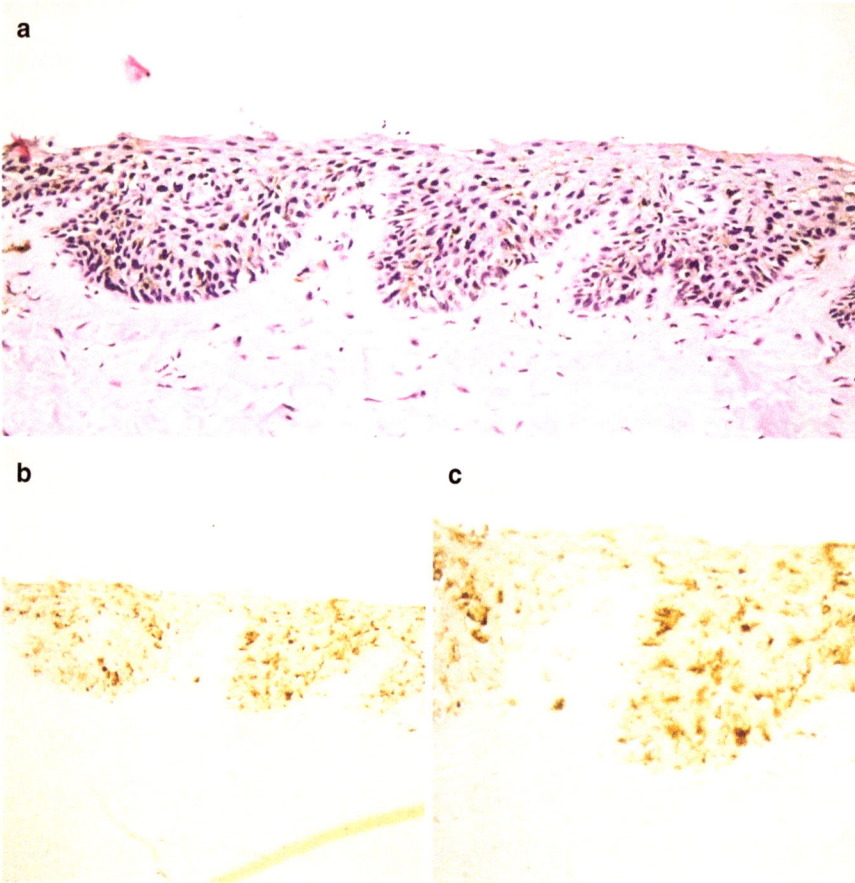

Fig. 20.3 Longitudinal melanonychia of the right index—histopathological aspect revealing: (**a**) cytonuclear atypia (hypertrophic, hyperchromatic, moderately pleomorphic nuclei) and the architectural anomalies (pagetoid ascension)—highly suggestive for in situ melanoma—hematoxylin eosin stain 200×; (**b**) significant pagetoid ascension and no dermal component—T311 stain 200× and (**c**) 400×

Diagnosis

Primary in situ non-ulcerated melanoma of the nail apparatus.

Discussion

Nail unit melanoma represents an uncommon subtype of acral melanoma, with a prevalence of 1–3% of all melanomas encountered in Caucasian population and 8–33% in non-Caucasians [1], being associated with poorer prognosis compared to other cutaneous melanoma types due to late diagnosis. The most frequent clinical presentation is represented by longitudinal melanonychia associated with Hutchinson sign, when the origin of the tumor is located in the nail matrix, while in the case of nail bed origin it presents as a nodule, with variable degrees of erythema, bleeding and ulceration [2]. Although longitudinal melanonychia located at a single digit in an adult patient bears a high index of nail unit melanoma suspicion, the accurate and early diagnosis can prove to be significantly difficult. Dermoscopy can be a useful tool when dealing with longitudinal melanonychia; pre-surgical dermoscopy helps choosing the proper biopsy area through examination of the distal nail edge—pigmentation of the upper half of the nail plate is a clue of proximal nail matrix origin, while pigmentation located in the lower half corresponds to distal nail matrix origin. On the other hand, intraoperative dermoscopy of the nail matrix, although is an invasive procedure, allows for a more accurate diagnosis, being useful in the differential diagnosis of longitudinal melanonychia and also helps guiding the proper biopsy site [3]. There are four intraoperative dermatoscopic patterns of the nail matrix: regular grey, regular brown, regular brown with globules/blotches and irregular, with the irregular one being associated with melanoma [4].

Although nail matrix biopsy remains the gold standard diagnostic approach for longitudinal melanonychia [5], its practical implementation can be limited by both physician's and patient's concerns regarding its invasive character and potential sequelae (pain, onychodystrophy) [6]. In order to help evaluating the risk-benefit ratio on proceeding with a biopsy of the nail matrix, Ohn et al. proposed an 8-point scoring model based on specific dermoscopic findings for differentiation between benign LM and subungual melanoma in situ (SMIS); the following five dermoscopic criteria were proposed to be checked when dealing with single digit longitudinal melanonychia in an adult patient: asymmetry and poorly defined borders of the pigmented band, multicolor pigmentation, width of the pigmented lesion equal or greater than 3 or 6 mm and the presence of Hutchison sign [6]. Although in this particular case, none of the five criteria were present in the early stages of the LM, dermoscopy guided matrix biopsy were performed.

Excisional biopsy—in which the lesion can be examined comprehensively—is recommended compared to punch biopsies, since the last might be associated to false-negative results determined by the limited tissue available for examination [3]; in most of the cases patients are reluctant in accepting the procedure. In our own experience, in other case of single digit LM of a young adult with worrisome clinical and dermoscopic characteristics, that agreed with total matrixectomy as a first diagnosis step, the pathology report showed benign findings (Fig. 20.4). In this regard, age may be important as well [7].

Some histopathological criteria for the diagnosis of in situ nail unit melanoma include an irregular distribution and asymmetry of melanocytes, increased intraepidermal and suprabasal melanocyte proliferation, tendency of nests fusions, atypical cells and lymphoid dermal inflammatory infiltrate; additionally, identification of just one melanocyte in the nail plate may be a sign of malignancy [5]. Complete surgical excision of the nail apparatus (including nail plate, nail bed and matrix) is recommended for in situ melanoma of the nail apparatus [8].

Fig. 20.4 Nail matrix nevus in a 24-year old male; clinical (**a**) and dermoscopy (**b**) aspect

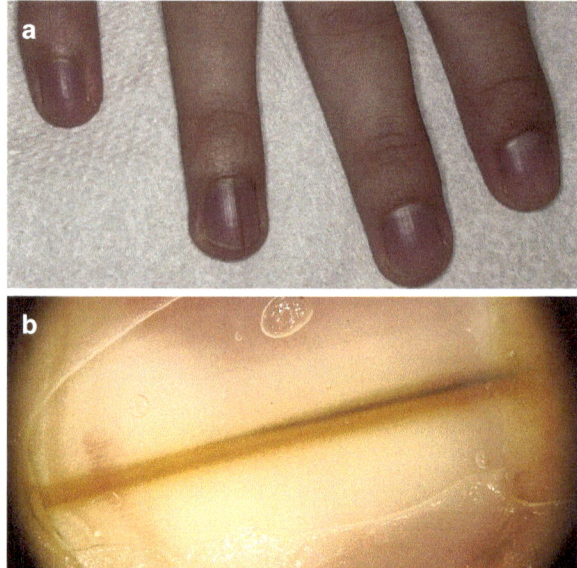

Melanonychia striata presents as a longitudinal streak of pigment that extends from the proximal nail fold to the distal margin of the nail plate and it can be determined by two main events: either activation or hyperplasia of melanocytes. Among the common causes of increased activity of melanocytes are darker skin phototypes, pregnancy, local repeated traumas, fungal or bacterial infections, drugs (sulfonamides, minocycline, azoles, antimalarial, chemotherapeutic agents), radiotherapy, inflammatory dermatological conditions (lichen planus, pustular psoriasis) or certain syndromes (Peutz-Jeghers, Laugier-Hunziker). Melanocytic hyperplasia associated with melanonychia striata can be encountered in nail matrix nevus, nail lentigo or nail unit melanoma [8, 9].

Onychomatricoma represents an uncommon benign fibroepitelial tumor of the nail matrix, in most cases presenting with xantonychia, longitudinal overcurvature and thickening of the nail plate; in rarer cases, it can associate longitudinal melanonychia, presenting as a polychromatic longitudinal band with Hutchinson sign, making the differential diagnosis with melanoma difficult. The histopathological features favoring pigmented onychomatricoma are represented by papillomatous matrix epithelium (presenting as "gloved-finger" digitations) and a fibrous dermal proliferation [10].

Subungual hematoma usually develops after local mechanical trauma (acute or chronic repeated) to the nail unit and it presents as a homogenous red-black discoloration of the nail plate, without any granules of melanin upon dermoscopy, evolving with a progressively distal dissolution as the nail grows. In unusual cases, subungual hemorrhage can originate in a nail matrix tumor, in which case it doesn't fade away as the nail grows; therefore, the presence of blood underneath the nail plate is not a specific clinical criteria for melanoma rule out [8].

Blue nevi of the nail matrix are not very common, with three distinct subtypes being described until now (common blue nevus or Jadassohn-Tièche type, cellular blue nevus and epitheloid blue nevus). It can present with multiple clinical pictures—ranging from longitudinal melanonychia to blue-black subungual nodule. The histopathological findings consistent with subungual blue nevi include normal nail plate and nail matrix, well-circumscribed collections of spindled cells that contain melanin granules, dermal pigment incontinence, free dermal and intracytoplasmic (within the epithelioid cells) melanin and a lack of atypical features (e.g. asymmetry, junctional proliferation of melanocytes, pagetoid extension, mitoses or cyto-architectural atypia). No treatment is neccessary; patients are being followed clinically and dermoscopically in order to identify any potential changes [11].

The histologic diagnosis of nail unit melanoma can prove difficult. Cytologic atypia can be subtle as melanocytes are often small with hyperchromatic and angulated nuclei. Features of nail unit melanoma may include multinucleated melanocytes, single cell predominance, irregular nests, confluence of melanocytes, prominent pagetoid spread and lichenoid inflammatory cell infiltrate. Nail fragments obtained as part of a diagnostic procedure in the nail unit should be submitted for evaluation and carefully inspected since nail unit epithelium comprising the melanocytic proliferation often remains attached. The presence of scattered melanocytes with large and hyperchromatic nuclei in a partial nail matrix biopsy is a diagnostic clue to nail unit melanoma in situ [12].

Key Points

- Nail unit melanoma is a rare type of acral melanoma, with poorer prognosis due to late diagnosis.
- Maintaining a high level of suspicion is very helpful.
- Dermoscopy represents a useful tool both for diagnosis and choosing the proper biopsy location, with intraoperative dermoscopy being more specific.
- Histopathological examination is the gold standard for nail unit melanoma diagnosis, with the total matrixectomy technique being suitable for a more accurate diagnosis. The timing for the procedure however needs to be very carefully chosen. Sometimes it may be delayed by the reluctance of both patients and specialists due to the invasiveness of the method and the prospect of permanent loss of the nail, especially if the clinical aspect does not fulfill any of the worrisome criteria and this may be the case in the very early stages of the adult single digit LM.
- Total surgical excision of the nail unit—plate, bed and matrix—represents the gold standard of treatment in cases of in situ nail unit melanoma.

References

1. Littleton TW, Murray PM, Baratz ME. Subungual melanoma. Orthop Clin North Am. 2019 Jul;50(3):357–66.
2. De Georgi V, Saggini A, Grazzini M, et al. Specific challenges in the management of subungual melanoma. Expert Rev Anticancer Ther. 2011;11(5):749–61.
3. Tosti A, Piraccini BM, de Farias DC. Dealing with melanonychia. Semin Cutan Med Surg. 2009;28(1):49–54.
4. Hirata SH, Yamada S, Enokihara MY, et al. Patterns of nail matrix and bed of longitudinal melanonychia by intraoperative dermoscopy. J Am Acad Dermatol. 2011;65(2):297–303.
5. Güneş P, Göktay F. Melanocytic lesions of the nail unit. Dermatopathology. 2018;5(3):98–107.
6. Ohn J, Jo G, Cho Y, Sheu SL, Cho KH, Mun JH. Assessment of a predictive scoring model for dermoscopy of subungual melanoma in situ. JAMA Dermatol. 2018;154(8):890–6.
7. Tosti A, Baran R, Piraccini BM, Cameli N, Fanti PA. Nail matrix nevi: a clinical and histopathologic study of twenty-two patients. J Am Acad Dermatol. 1996;34:765–71.
8. Braun RP, et al. Diagnosis and management of nail pigmentations. J Am Acad Dermatol. 2007;56(5):835–47.
9. Leung AK, Lam JM, Leong KF, Sergi CM. Melanonychia striata: clarifying behind the Black Curtain. A review on clinical evaluation and management of the 21st century. Int J Dermatol. 2019;58(11):1239–45.
10. Isales MC, Haugh AM, Bubley J, et al. Pigmented onychomatricoma: a rare mimic of subungual melanoma. Clin Exp Dermatol. 2018;43(5):623–6.
11. Smith DF, Morgan MB, Bettencourt MS. Longitudinal Melanonychia-Quiz case. Arch Dermatol. 2003;139(9):1209–14.
12. Gatica-Torres M, Nelson CA, Lipoff JB, Miller CJ, Rubin AI. Nail clipping with onychomycosis and surprise clue to the diagnosis of nail unit melanoma. J Cutan Pathol. 2018;45:803–6.

Chapter 21
A Female Patient with the Small Pigmented Lesion

Jelena Stojkovic-Filipovic and Martina Bosic

An 58-year-old female patient came for a preventive exam in a screening campaign for early diagnosis of melanoma. She pointed out the lesion on her arm, unable to determine the duration of the lesion. Her personal and family history for cutaneous malignances were negative. Previously, in her youth, she had unprotected UV exposure during summer months. She was otherwise healthy, without chronic conditions, and she was not taking any medication.

Clinical exam revealed a small, intensively pigmented, asymmetric lesion, four millimeters in diameter, on the lateral part of the left upper arm (Figs. 21.1 and 21.2).

Based on the case description and the photographs, what is your diagnosis?

1. Seborrheic keratosis
2. Pigmented Basal Cell Carcinoma
3. Melanoma
4. Pigmented Actinic keratosis
5. Melanocytic nevus

Dermoscopy showed chaotic pigmented lesion, with mainly eccentric structureless pattern eccentric black area, and central gray-brown hue. In the center of the lesion, asymmetric dark brown unequally thick lines were noted. Segmental brown radial lines were noticed at the periphery of the lesion as well as brown dots in asymmetric fashion (Fig. 21.3).

J. Stojkovic-Filipovic (✉)
Clinic of Dermatovenereology, Clinical Centre of Serbia, Belgrade, Serbia

Department of Dermatovenereology, School of Medicine, University of Belgrade, Belgrade, Serbia

M. Bosic
Institute of Pathology, School of Medicine, University of Belgrade, Belgrade, Serbia

T. Lotti et al. (eds.), *Clinical Cases in Melanoma*, Clinical Cases in Dermatology, https://doi.org/10.1007/978-3-030-50820-3_21

Fig. 21.1 Clinical presentation: small, pigmented papule on the upper arm

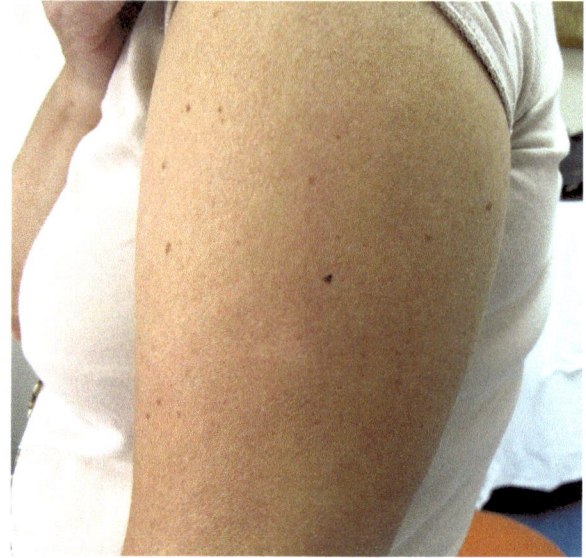

Fig. 21.2 Clinical presentation: close up of slightly elevated pigmented lesion

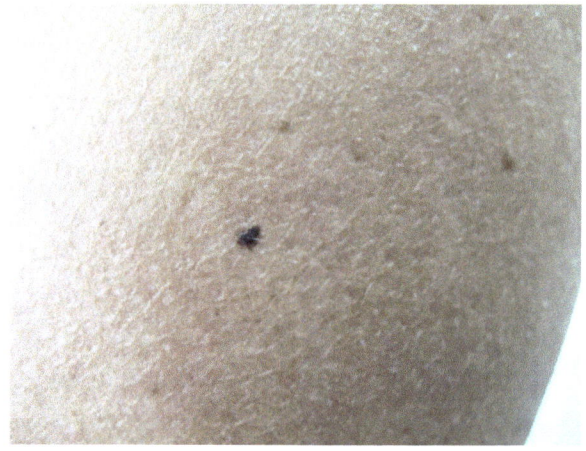

The wide excision was performed and histopathological exam revealed atypical epithelioid melanocytes forming small irregular nests in epidermis or in focal lentiginous arrangement. Papillary dermis showed light-moderate infiltration with lymphocytes and melanophages without atypical melanocytes (Fig. 21.4).

Diagnosis

Superficial spreading melanoma in situ.

Fig. 21.3 Dermoscopy features

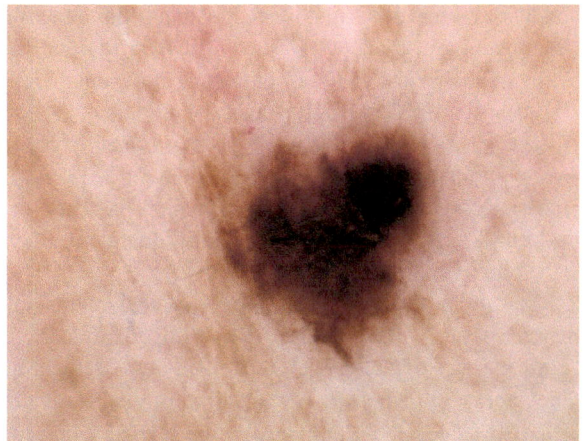

Fig. 21.4 Histopathological findings

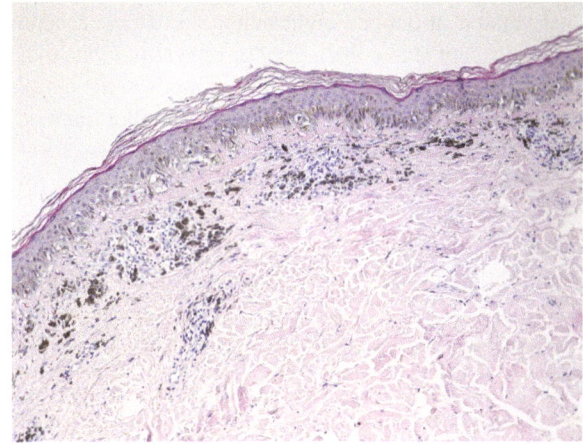

Discussion

Melanoma, a malignant tumor that arises from melanocytes, most commonly has cutaneous origin, although it can arise on mucosal surfaces, eye, and leptomeninges [1]. It is one of the most common forms of cancer in young adults and due to its metastatic potential leads to more than 90% of skin cancer related deaths [1]. Early detection of melanoma is crucial to improve survival in patients with melanoma.

The ABCDs rule (**A**symmetry, **B**order irregularity, **C**olor variegation, and **D**iameter > 6 mm) was proposed as a mnemonic guide for the public awareness and clinical diagnosis of cutaneous melanoma [1]. Latter, "**E**", for **E**volving, has been added to highlight the importance of a changing of the lesion. The ABCDE guide has been used by dermatologists worldwide, and has been suggested to patients for self-examination. The presence of very small (≤6 mm diameter) cutaneous melanomas has prompted the reconsideration of the role of diameter, thus change of the meaning of the letter D, from *diameter* to *dark*, has been proposed [2]. Current clinical definition of small-diameter melanoma, i.e. melanoma not fulfilling the 'D'criterion of the ABCD(E) clinical alphabet ('D' less than 6 mm in its maximum diameter) is contemplated, since significant proportion of melanomas may be smaller than 6 mm in early stages, at the time of diagnosis. Some studies considered the concept of 'micro-melanoma' which has been defined on clinical grounds as ≤3 mm in width, different to the traditional definition of small-diameter melanoma (≤6 mm in diameter) [3].

In situ and early invasive cutaneous melanoma can be subtle in appearance and not necessarily meet previously mentioned clinical criteria [4]. The use of dermoscopy in screening campaigns led to an improvement in diagnostic accuracy in early melanoma, allowing the visualization of diagnostic criteria not visible to the naked eye [5]. Since early-stage melanomas are often curable by surgical excision, it is of great importance to diagnose them as early as possible. The chaos and clues algorithm is relatively new, and it is a condensed variant of pattern analysis. In its original version, it defined eight melanoma clues: eccentric structureless zones of any color (except skin color), gray or blue structures, black dots or clods in the periphery, segmental radial lines or pseudopods at the periphery, white lines, thick reticular lines, polymorphous vessels, and parallel lines on the ridges (for acral lesions) [5]. Melanomas in situ are usually chaotic, but chaos alone is commonly not sufficient to diagnose pigmented malignant neoplasms. Most in situ melanomas show at least two clues to malignancy [4]. In a direct comparison of melanoma in situ with atypical ("dysplastic") nevi, five variables are identified (atypical network, regression >50%, irregular hyperpigmented areas, angulated lines, and prominent skin markings). The presence of irregular hyperpigmented areas and the presence of prominent skin markings proved to be particularly useful clues to differentiate melanoma in situ from atypical nevi [6].

References

1. Bolognia J, Scaffer JV, Cerroni L. Dermatology. St Louis: Mosby Elsevier; 2018.
2. Abbasi NR, Shaw HM, Rigel DS, et al. Early diagnosis of cutaneous melanoma: revisiting the ABCD criteria. JAMA. 2004;292(22):2771–6.
3. Bono A, Tolomio E, Trincone S, et al. Micro- melanoma detection: a clinical study on 206 consecutive cases of pigmented skin lesions with a diameter ≤3 mm. Br J Dermatol. 2006;155:570.
4. Weber P, Tschandl P, Sinz C, Kittler H. Dermatoscopy of neoplastic skin lesions: recent advances, updates, and revisions. Curr Treat Options Oncol. 2018;19(11):56.
5. Kittler H, editor. Dermatoscopy: pattern analysis of pigmented and non-pigmented lesions. 2nd ed. Vienna: Facultas Publishing AG; 2016.
6. Lallas A, Longo C, Manfredini M, Benati E, Babino G, Chinazzo C, et al. Accuracy of dermoscopic criteria for the diagnosis of melanoma in situ. JAMA Dermatol. 2018;154(4):414–9.

Chapter 22
An Elderly Female with a Vaginal Mass

Ritu Swali, Rohit Gupta, Madeline Frizzell, and Stephen K. Tyring

An 85-year-old Caucasian female with no past medical history presented to the emergency room complaining of abnormal vaginal bleeding for the past year. She stated that the bleeding had been accompanied by bilateral lower extremity edema and fatigue. On physical examination, there was a malodorous, hyperpigmented, hemorrhagic mass protruding from the vagina (Fig. 22.1), along with left inguinal lymphadenopathy.

Based on the case description and photograph, what is your diagnosis?
1. Poorly differentiated squamous cell carcinoma
2. Extramammary Paget disease
3. Vaginal primary malignant melanoma
4. Leiomyosarcoma

   Due to anemia and urethral obstruction from the mass, the patient was hospitalized for further work-up. A pelvic ultrasound was performed, revealing a vaginal mass measuring 11.9 cm × 6.7 cm × 10.6 cm. Ultrasound-guided inguinal lymph node biopsy showed neoplastic cells with nuclear hyperchromasia, enlargement,

R. Swali (✉)
Center for Clinical Studies, Houston, TX, USA

R. Gupta
Baylor College of Medicine, Houston, TX, USA
e-mail: rohit.gupta@bcm.edu

M. Frizzell
Texas A&M University College of Medicine, Houston, TX, USA

S. K. Tyring
Department of Dermatology, Center for Clinical Studies, McGovern Medical School at UT Houston Health Sciences Center, Houston, TX, USA
e-mail: Styring@ccstexas.com

T. Lotti et al. (eds.), *Clinical Cases in Melanoma*,
Clinical Cases in Dermatology, https://doi.org/10.1007/978-3-030-50820-3_22

Fig. 22.1 An 85-year-old female presented with a 1-year history of abnormal vaginal bleeding

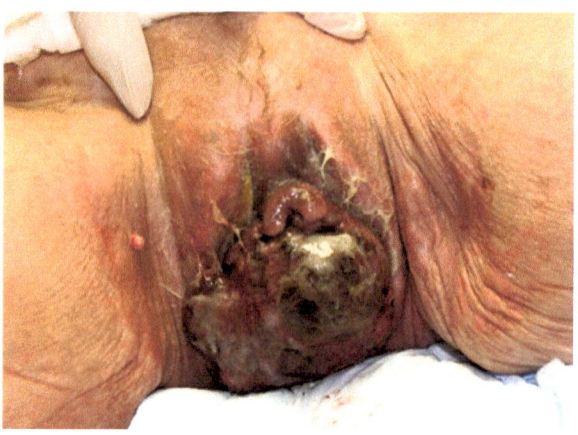

and pleomorphism. Additionally, a core biopsy of the vaginal mass demonstrated pleomorphic neoplastic cells with associated necrosis and fibrosis. Immunostaining was positive for MART-1, CD117, Vimentin, and S100.

Diagnosis Vaginal Primary Metastatic Malignant Melanoma.

Discussion

Vaginal primary malignant melanoma (VPMM) is one of many primary mucosal melanomas, which are characterized by aberrant melanocyte proliferation in the mucosal linings of urogenital, respiratory, and gastrointestinal tracts. VPMM is exceedingly rare, constituting approximately 0.5% of melanomas and 3% of vaginal malignancies [1, 2].

While ultraviolet radiation is known to play a role in the development of melanomas, the exact etiology of those that develop in non-sun exposed regions, including the vaginal mucosa, is unclear [1]. VPMM arises from aberrant melanocytes found in the vaginal basal epidermis [3]. The pathogenesis of this tumor is associated with genetic mutations in B-Raf proto-oncogene serine/threonine kinase (*BRAF*) and *KIT,* with the latter being more specific to mucosal melanomas [3, 4]. High expression of topoisomerase IIα (TOP2A), PD-1, and PD-L1 is commonly noted [4].

The disease is usually diagnosed in postmenopausal women, with no ethnic or socioeconomic predilections [1, 3]. Classic presentation of VPMM is vaginal pruritus, discharge, and bleeding; however, many patients are asymptomatic. Larger tumors may be visible on external genital exam at presentation. Diagnosis is made by manual and ultrasound-guided examination of the pelvis, with subsequent CT or MRI to locate the primary site. The tumor typically is a polypoid and ulcerated vaginal mass, often found in the lower one-third and anterior wall of the vagina [1].

Because of the late presentation of the tumor and the rich vascular and lymphatic network of the vaginal mucosa, VPMM is often a very aggressive malignancy, with approximately one-third of patients having lymph node metastases at presentation [1]. Although no staging system has been a useful prognosticator, historically, tumor size (<3 cm versus ≥3 cm) has been the most important prognostic factor, with larger tumors associated with worse outcomes [1]. The five-year survival rate of VPMM ranges from 8.4% to 27%, whereas cutaneous melanomas can have rates as high as 81% [1, 3].

Current therapeutic modalities include wide local excision, radical surgery, chemotherapy, immunotherapy, combination therapy, or palliative care. Surgical excision has been the most promising treatment; radiation therapy is often used as adjuvant therapy for tumors larger than 3 cm or postoperatively in cases involving local pelvic metastases [1, 3]. Chemotherapy with dacarbazine and immunotherapy with interferon and interleukin-2 have been used in advanced stages of the disease with limited response [4]. Similarly, case reports of anti-PD-1 agents (pembrolizumab, nivolumab) and anti-CTLA 4 agents (ipilimumab) have documented limited efficacy [5].

Poorly differentiated squamous cell carcinoma can clinically appear to be similar to this exophytic, ulcerative tumor. There are two types of squamous carcinoma in the genital region. Basaloid and warty carcinomas (30% of cases) are related to infection with human papilloma virus, while keratinizing squamous cell carcinoma (70% of cases) involve chronic epithelial irritation, lichen sclerosis or squamous cell hyperplasia [6]. Vulvectomy and lymphadenectomy with adjuvant radiation are the standard treatment regimen utilized to ensure good long-term survival [7].

Extramammary Paget disease may also mimic VPMM, but the lesions usually present as a pruritic, red, crusted area on the labia majora. Paget disease consists of intraepithelial malignant cells, which are larger and have paler cytoplasm than surrounding keratocytes. However, unlike Paget disease of the nipple, Paget disease of the vulva is not associated with underlying cancer and is confined to the epidermis. Treatment consists of wide local excision [7].

Due to the location of the lesion, leiomyosarcoma is included in the differential. It is an uncommon malignant neoplasm that grows as a bulky, fleshy mass with areas of hemorrhage and necrosis. Peak incidence for these tumors is between 40 and 60 years in either pre or post menopausal women. These are aggressive tumors that often recur after surgery and more than half will hematogenously metastasize to the lungs, bones or brain. Distinction can easily be made with histopathological examination of the affected tissue [7].

Based on the patient's medical history, appearance of the lesion, and histopathological findings, the diagnosis of VPMM was made. Although surgical resection and chemotherapy are considered first-line treatments for VPMM, the patient was unable to tolerate these due to frailty. Instead, a six-week course of radiation was initiated to shrink the mass, and the patient was transferred to a skilled nursing facility where she remained neurologically intact, but bedridden. Ultimately, the patient was placed on hospice care and died of her cancer.

Key Points
- Vaginal primary malignant melanoma is a rare aggressive primary mucosal melanoma with poor prognosis.
- Typical presentation of this tumor is vaginal pruritus, discharge, and bleeding.
- Mainstay of treatment is surgical excision with adjuvant radiation.

References

1. Androutsopoulos G, Terzakis E, Ioannidou G, Tsamandas A, Decavalas G. Vaginal primary malignant melanoma: a rare and aggressive tumor. Case Rep Obstet Gynecol. 2013;2013:137908.
2. Schmidt M, Honig A, Schwab M, Adam P, Dietl J. Primary vaginal melanoma: a case report and literature review. Eur J Gynaecol Oncol. 2008;29(3):285–8.
3. Kalampokas E, Kalampokas T, Damaskos C. Primary vaginal melanoma, a rare and aggressive entity. A case report and review of the literature. In Vivo. 2017;31(1):133–9.
4. Hou JY, Baptiste C, Hombalegowda RB, et al. Vulvar and vaginal melanoma: a unique subclass of mucosal melanoma based on a comprehensive molecular analysis of 51 cases compared with 2253 cases of nongynecologic melanoma. Cancer. 2017;123(8):1333–44.
5. Indini A, Di guardo L, Cimminiello C, Lorusso D, Raspagliesi F, Del vecchio M. Investigating the role of immunotherapy in advanced/recurrent female genital tract melanoma: a preliminary experience. J Gynecol Oncol. 2019;30(6):e94.
6. Robbins SL, Cotran RS, Aster JC, Kumar V, Abbas AK. Robbins and Cotran pathologic basis of disease. 9th ed. Philadelphia: Elsevier; 2015.
7. Puri S, Asotra S. Primary vaginal malignant melanoma: a rare entity with review of literature. J Cancer Res Ther. 2019;15(6):1392–4.

Chapter 23
A Dark Spot in a Subject with Renal Carcinoma

I. Condrat, A. Tataru, and D. Tataru

A 43-year-old man presented to our clinic with high anxiety regarding a melanocytic lesion on his posterior thorax (Fig. 23.1). The lesion was asymptomatic and the patient was unaware of it. Presumably, the lesion was unchanged over the past years. The location on the posterior thorax made it hard for the patient to keep an eye on its evolution. A previous visit to the endocrinologist who saw the lesion urged the patient to visit the dermatology clinic.

Clinical examination and history revealed no risk factors, no history of sunburns and no prior history of skin cancer. His family history noted few and far relatives with variable malignancies and cancer diagnosis. On clinical examination, no constitutional symptoms, cardiac, respiratory or abdominal complaints were present. Full physical exam showed no enlarged lymph nodes and no other pathologic or worrisome skin changes.

Moreover, multiple melanocytic nevi were present and disseminated on the posterior and anterior thorax, upper and lower limbs and on the face, without any possible malignant changes on dermoscopy.

Based on the case description and the photograph, what is your diagnosis?

1. Melanocytic nevus
2. Melanoma in situ
3. Superficial spreading melanoma
4. Reed Nevus (pigmented spindle cell nevus)

I. Condrat · A. Tataru (✉)
Department of Dermatology, Iuliu Hatieganu University of Medicine and Pharmacy, Cluj-Napoca, Romania

D. Tataru
Department of Internal Medicine, Iuliu Hatieganu University of Medicine and Pharmacy, Cluj-Napoca, Romania

T. Lotti et al. (eds.), *Clinical Cases in Melanoma*, Clinical Cases in Dermatology, https://doi.org/10.1007/978-3-030-50820-3_23

107

Fig. 23.1 Dermoscopy
aspect of the suspect lesion

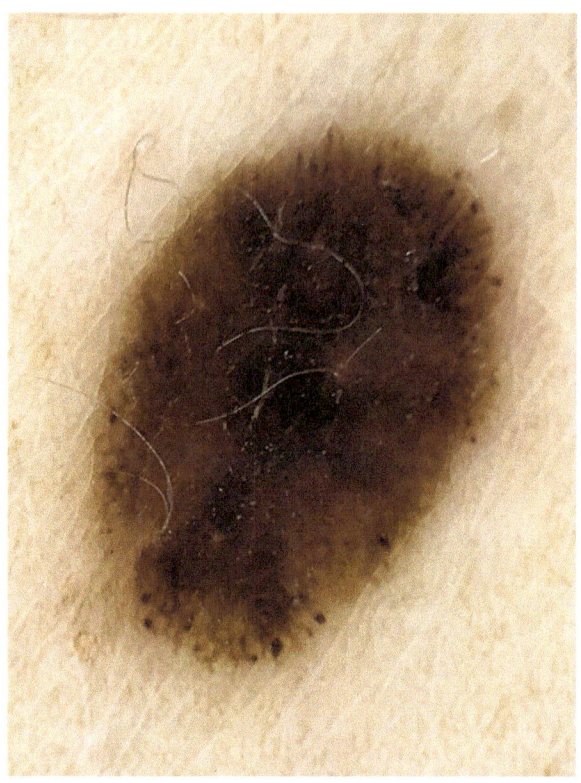

After clinical and dermoscopy examination of the lesion in Fig. 23.1, an excisional biopsy was performed with 0.3 mm margins in healthy tissue and the lesion was sent to pathology for examination. Histopathological exam revealed a proliferation of melanocytes in the junctional area with marked atypical nuclei and a pagetoid extension of these cells. Ulceration was absent, there was no angiolymphatic extension and of high importance was the lack of melanocytic atypical cells in the dermis, therefore revealing an in-situ melanoma.

Primary treatment for in situ melanoma includes wide excision and the recommended clinical margins are 0.5–1.0 cm [1]. Wide excision was performed, with negative margins.

Diagnosis

In situ malignant melanoma on the skin.

Discussion

According to the last guidelines in cutaneous melanoma, for stage 0 melanoma in situ routine imaging or other lab test are not recommended and imaging is required only to evaluate specific signs or symptoms [1]. However, due to the high anxiety of the patient, nodal basin ultrasonography was performed after the primary excision and a pathological abnormality was revealed on the left kidney, raising the suspicion of a renal tumour. A urology consult and CT were indicated to further evaluate the lesion.

For the renal tumour, a chest/abdominal/pelvic CT was performed, which revealed a round-oval lesion on the inferior and posterior pole of the left kidney, well defined, inhomogeneous, partially extrarenal. It extended up until the caliceal groups inferior, but without invasion. The tumour was excised, and the histopathology exam showed a renal cell carcinoma, with solid architecture and large clear cells, a variant named chromophobe. Final diagnosis was melanoma in situ, a blue nevus and a clear cell renal carcinoma.

This is an unusual case of melanoma in situ in a young adult, with no risk factors, with a synchronous renal carcinoma. Such rare cases are presented scarcely in the literature and an underlying germline BRCA2 mutation was postulated in a 54-year-old woman with nodular melanoma and clear cell renal carcinoma after a next generation sequencing panel of 25 hereditary cancer genes was performed [2]. The 54 years old woman was heterogenous in BRCA2 gene, with a frame shift mutation leading to a possible premature termination codon, and a missense mutation with uncertain significance. The gene BRCA (breast cancer susceptibility gene) are tumour suppression genes that maintain the integrity of the genome and mutations in the genes lead to various types of cancers, from the main breast cancers, to pancreatic, prostate or gastric cancers [2]. Furthermore, a study that researched hereditary background of renal cancer in Denmark noted that another renal cell carcinoma susceptibility gene, called BAP1, which regulates pathways in cell cycles, is known to predispose to cutaneous melanoma [3]. Kim and colleagues found a strong association between the diagnosis of melanoma and renal cell carcinoma and noted that this phenomenon could be either due to more thorough and frequent examinations in a patient after an initial cancer, due to underlying immunocompromised conditions or due to therapies for the first cancer diagnosis [4].

Considering all data, we aim to support previous studies that a genetic predisposition is necessary for the development of two synchronous tumours such as renal cell carcinoma and melanoma. Modernised genetic testing is required in patients who present with atypical disease course or who have unique features. Further genetic studies are mandatory to elucidate the pathogenetic pathways.

For our patient a multidisciplinary team was set in place, with a urologist and an oncologist to further follow up the patient. No genetic testing has been done until present. From a dermatological point of view, annually follow up with clinical and dermoscopic evaluation is recommended for all the melanocytic lesions and for the evaluation of the postoperative scar. The patient was instructed to avoid sun exposure and use creams with high sun protection factors.

Key Points

Malignant melanoma arising in a relatively young patient without any known risk factors suggests a genetic background.

The synchronous presentation of a two different and aggressive types of cancers in the same patient should be investigated for genetic mutations, at least for BRCA2 and BAP1 genes.

References

1. Coit DG, Thompson JA, Albertini MR, et al. Cutaneous melanoma, version 2.2019, NCCN clinical practice guidelines in oncology. J Natl Compr Cancer Netw. 2019;17(4):367–402. https://doi.org/10.6004/jnccn.2019.0018.
2. Snow A, Ricker C. Two synchronous malignancies: nodular melanoma and renal cell carcinoma in a patient with an underlying germline BRCA2 mutation. BMJ Case Reports. 2019;12:e227625.
3. Christensen MB, Wadt K, Jensen UB, Lautrup CK, Bojesen A, Krogh LN, et al. Exploring the hereditary background of renal cancer in Denmark. PLoS One. 2019;14(4):e0215725. https://doi.org/10.1371/journal.pone.0215725.
4. Kim K, Chung TH, Etzel CJ, Kim J, Ryu H, et al. Association between melanoma and renal-cell carcinoma for sequential diagnoses: a single-center retrospective study. Cancer Epidemiol. 2018 Dec;57:80–4. https://doi.org/10.1016/j.canep.2018.10.003.

Chapter 24
Cutaneous Melanoma from Anterior Thorax: A Case Report

Florin Ciprian Bujoreanu, Diana Sabina Radaschin, Lawrence Chukwudi Nwabudike, and Alin Laurentiu Tatu

We present the case of a 51-year-old male, referred to our clinic for the presence of a pigmented mole, located on the anterior thorax. It measured 1.4 × 1.2 cm, was asymptomatic, with no bleeding or ulceration. The lesion developed on a preexisting nevus and the patient claims that it had grown continuously in the last 2 years (Fig. 24.1). The dermatoscopic evaluation raised the suspicion of melanoma (Fig. 24.2). To confirm the diagnosis, he underwent an excisional biopsy, which was completed by sentinel lymph node biopsy. Histology confirmed the diagnosis of malignant melanoma, with Breslow thickness of 0.6 mm, Clark level II, without a vertical growth phase, mitosis, lymphatic or vascular invasion (Fig. 24.3). There was no involvement of the lymph nodes seen.

F. C. Bujoreanu
"Dunărea de Jos" University, Galati, Romania

Dermatology Department, Infectious Diseases Clinical Hospital "St. Parascheva", Galati, Romania

D. S. Radaschin
Dermatology Department, Infectious Diseases Clinical Hospital "St. Parascheva", Galati, Romania

Faculty of Medicine and Pharmacy/Clinical Department, Dermatology, "Dunărea de Jos" University, Galati, Romania

L. C. Nwabudike
N. Paulescu Institute, Bucharest, Romania

A. L. Tatu (✉)
Faculty of Medicine and Pharmacy/Clinical Department, Dermatology, Medical and Pharmaceutical Research Unit, Competitive, Interdisciplinary Research Integrated Platform "Dunărea de Jos", ReForm-UDJG "Dunărea de Jos" University, Infectious Diseases Clinical Hospital "St. Parascheva" Dermatalogy, Galati, Romania

© The Editor(s) (if applicable) and The Author(s), under exclusive license to   111
Springer Nature Switzerland AG 2020
T. Lotti et al. (eds.), *Clinical Cases in Melanoma*,
Clinical Cases in Dermatology, https://doi.org/10.1007/978-3-030-50820-3_24

Fig. 24.1 Clinical aspect of the lesion. Pigmented melanocytic tumor situated on the anterior thorax of the patient

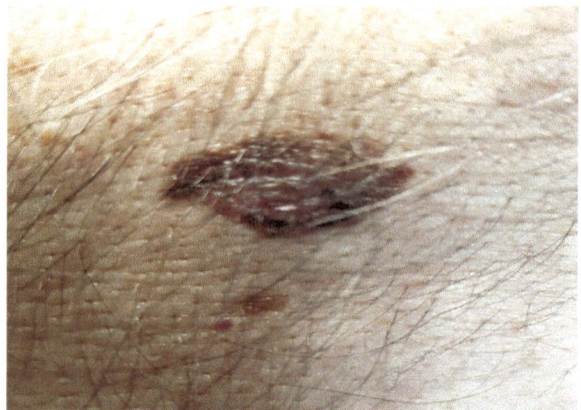

Fig. 24.2 Dermoscopic aspect of the lesion. A pigmented, asymmetric, with uneven borders, with multiple colours, with a diameter of about 12 mm, superficial spreading melanoma, which has grown continuously in the last 2 years

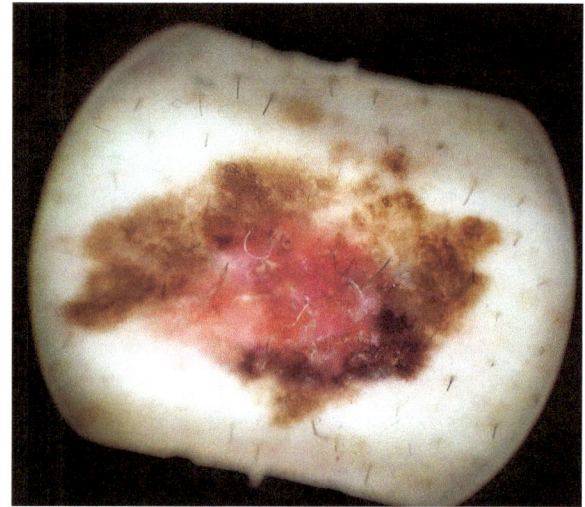

Based on the case description and the photograph, what is your diagnosis?

- Basal cell carcinoma (BCC)
- Seborrheic keratosis
- Dermatofibroma
- Traumatized or irritated naevus

Diagnosis

Slow growing melanoma with a Breslow of 0.6 mm.

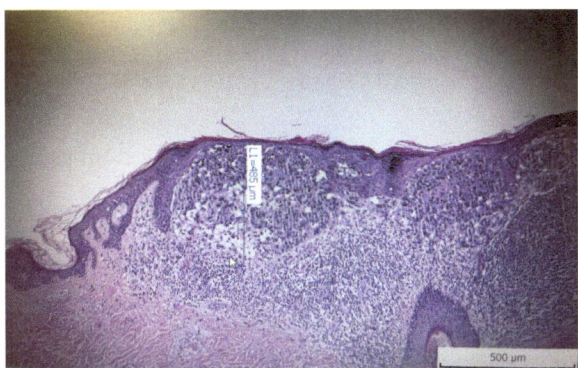

Fig. 24.3 Section showing histological features of malignant melanoma. Paraffin sections stained with Haematoxylin—Eosin showed features of malignant melanoma—Large cells with pleomorphic, hyperchromatic nuclei with prominent nucleoli and moderate amount of cytoplasm. No mitoses were seen per high power field

Discussion

Melanoma, also known as malignant melanoma, is a type of cancer that develops from the pigment-containing cells known as melanocytes. It attracts a great deal of attention because it is often lethal. It is considered to be the most dangerous type of skin cancer [1].

Melanoma is more common in men than women. However, it accounts for less than 5% of skin cancers.

Cutaneous melanoma currently represents a public health problem of worldwide importance.

Melanomas are usually caused by DNA damage resulting from exposure to ultraviolet light. Melanoma can also be located in skin areas with little skin exposure (mouth, palms, genital areas, soles) [2].

The ultraviolet radiation from tanning beds increases the risk of melanoma. The International Agency for Research on Cancer finds that people who begin using tanning devices before the age of 30 years are 75% more likely to develop melanoma. Exposure to ultraviolet radiation (UVA and UVB) is one of the major contributors to the development of melanoma. The risk of developing a malignant melanoma is highest in those with congenital melanocytic naevi, atypical naevi. Approximately 30% of melanoma cases appear on a pre-existing nevus [3].

Cutaneous melanoma is one of the most aggressive forms of cancer and one of the leading causes of oncological mortality through metastasis.

Early detection is the key to a better prognosis. Although melanoma may present characteristic features, dermoscopy should be used to clarify the differential diagnosis of pigmented lesions. The characteristic features include an atypical pigmented network, irregular brown-black dots/globules, streaks and pigmentation with multiple colours distributed asymmetrically. The blue-whitish veil and polymorphic vessels are common in invasive forms of melanoma [4].

Key Points
- Cutaneous melanoma is the leading cause of death from skin cancer, and it is considered a public health problem.
- In high risk patients, and in patients with atypical mole syndrome, the detection of changes in the lesions or newly appeared lesions by follow-up examination with digital dermatoscopy or total-body.
- Dermatoscopy is useful in prevention and early detection of cutaneous melanoma.

References

1. Leiter U, Garbe C. Epidemiology of melanoma and nonmelanoma skin cancer-the role of sunlight. Adv Exp Med Biol. 2008;624:89–103.
2. Eggermont AM, Spatz A, Robert C. Cutaneous melanoma. Lancet. 2014;383(9919):816–27.
3. Garbe C, Peris K, Hauschild A, Saiag P, Middleton M, Spatz A, et al. Diagnosis and treatment of melanoma: European consensus-based interdisciplinary guideline. Eur J Cancer. 2010;46(2):270–83.
4. Sewon K. Fitzpatrick's dermatology, 9th ed., 2-volume set, 8th Edition, chapter 124. Cutaneous melanoma; 2019.

Chapter 25
An Acral Spot in a 73-Year-Old Male

Ionela Manole, Alexandra-Irina Butacu, Sabina Zurac, and George-Sorin Tiplica

A 73-year-old male with no significant pathological history, presented in the Dermatology clinic with a melanotic lesion located on the right hallux, with involvement of the nail bed (Fig. 25.1). The lesion had a history of 12 months, with initial location on the distal phalanx and progressive change in size and color. On physical examination, the patient presented an irregular dark-brown pigmented patch, with superficial ulceration located on the distal phalanx of the right hallux (Fig. 25.2), with involvement of the nail, associating nail plate destruction. The patient reported minor bleeding in case of light trauma and no other associated symptoms. There was no evidence of clinically apparent lymph node metastasis. Initially, the patient refused surgical excision and a lesional imprint histology was performed which was not specific, revealing an inflammatory process. After one month, during the follow-up, it was noticed the extent of the pigmentary lesion and the patient underwent a wide local excision of the tumor in the Dermatology department. He was referred to the Oncology Department where it was performed hallux amputation and it was prescribed the therapy designed for his disease stage.

Histopathological examination revealed architectural asymmetric melanocytic proliferation with ulceration, with predominant development at the dermo-epidermic junction and intra-epidermic level; moderate cyto-nuclear pleomorphism. In the papillary dermis has been identified invasion of tumoral cells, in the form of nests and solitary cells, without mitotic activity (Fig. 25.3). Immunohistochemical examination of biopsied tissue sections showed positive staining for melanoma associated antigens using the antibodies HMB-45 (Fig. 25.4).

I. Manole · A.-I. Butacu · G.-S. Tiplica (✉)
2nd Department of Dermatology, Colentina Clinical Hospital, "Carol Davila" University of Medicine and Pharmacy, Bucharest, Romania

S. Zurac
Department of Pathology, Colentina Clinical Hospital, Bucharest, Romania

T. Lotti et al. (eds.), *Clinical Cases in Melanoma*, Clinical Cases in Dermatology, https://doi.org/10.1007/978-3-030-50820-3_25

Fig. 25.1 Ulcerated
melanotic lesion located on
the right hallux, with
involvement of the nail bed

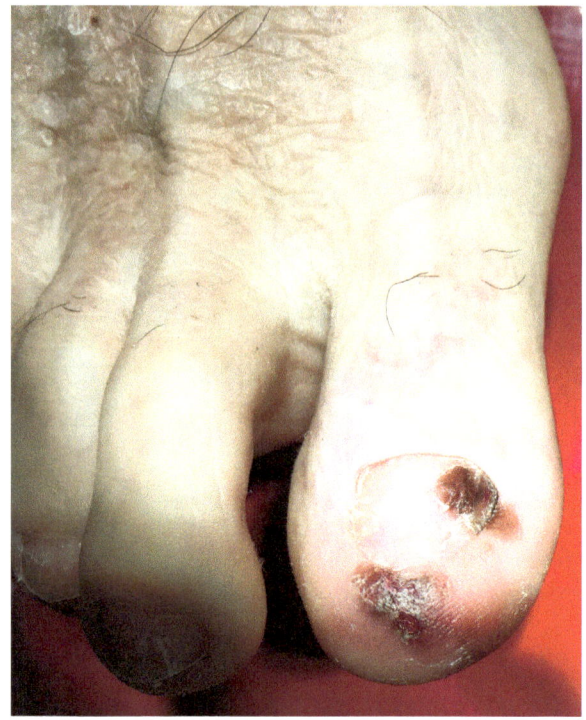

Based on the case description and the photograph, what is your diagnosis?

- Subungual haematoma
- Kaposi sarcoma
- Non-healing ulcer
- Onychomycosis

Diagnosis

Ulcerated acral lentiginous melanoma (ALM) with perineural and reticular dermis
invasion, Breslow index of 1.5 mm, Clark level IV (pT2bNM)

Discussions

ALM represents approximately 5% of all melanomas in white patients and the most
common melanoma subtype found in dark-skinned and Asian populations [1]. As
described by Reed, ALM develops in the acral regions of the body, particularly the
palms, soles, sometimes with nail involvement and is characterized by its lentiginous

Fig. 25.2 Ulcerated
melanotic lesion located on
the right hallux

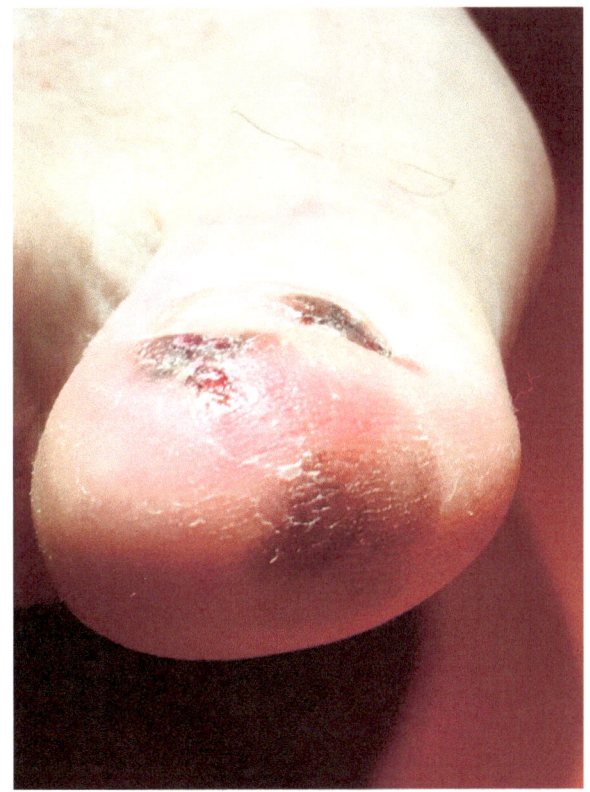

Fig. 25.3 Histopath-
ological examination
showing melanocyte
proliferation composed of
polyhedral cells with
pagetoid intraepidermal
infiltration (haematoxylin
eosin stain ×100)

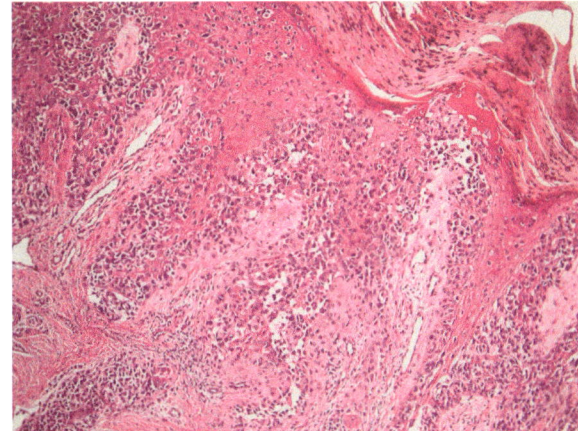

Fig. 25.4 HMB45 positive
staining of tumoral cells

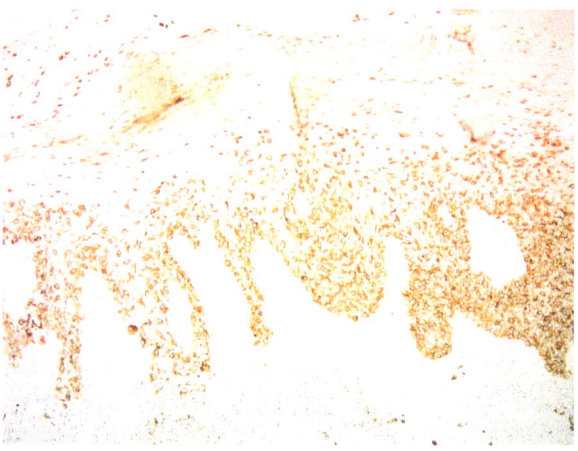

(radial) growth phase [2]. It can develop within an existing melanocytic nevus or may be related with different other causes such as trauma, environmental factors, exposure to chemical substances (e.g. agricultural chemicals), smoking or genetic factors [3]. ALM tends to have a poor prognosis due to the advanced stage in the moment of presentation, frequently as a consequence of delay diagnosis. The most common challenges in diagnosis are represented by tumor hidden location and similarity with other conditions such as non-healing wounds, paronychia, diabetic ulcers, warts, fungal infections, pyogenic granulomas or hematoma [4]. Wide local excision to achieve negative margins represents the conventional treatment in patients with ALM, followed by chemotherapy, immunotherapy or biologic treatment. Significant prognostic factors in patients with ALM are represented by advanced age, the presence of ulceration, tumor thickness and tumor spread in the moment of diagnosis [5].

Subungual haematoma is a condition frequently considered in the presence of a change in the nail color, often difficult to differentiate from acral melanoma even when analyzed by dermoscopy. It generally appears as a consequence of a direct local trauma or due to repetitive injury during sport activities. It is important to notice that in the subungual haematoma the pigment rarely extends outside the nail bed and generally clears proximally as the nail grows. The presence of the pigment on the nail folds and the heterogeneous distribution in both the longitudinal and transverse axes of the nail are useful hints that support the diagnosis of acral melanoma [6].

Kaposi sarcoma (KS) is a low-grade vascular tumor with herpesvirus type 8 playing a fundamental role in its development. Lesions present as purplish, reddish blue or dark brown/black macules, patches, nodules or plaques on the lower extremities, with an unchanged evolution for months, and frequently bleed. In patients with single lesions, ALM should be ruled out as possible cause of presentation. Histopathological examination is extremely important for the differential diagnosis with other malignant diseases, such as melanoma. The histology differs based on the disease's stage and consists in highlighting the proliferation of blood vessels in the dermis and subcutis and a variable chronic inflammatory infiltrate composed of lymphocytes, plasma cells, and dendritic cells [7].

Non-healing ulcers are commonly associated with certain medical conditions such as diabetes mellitus, chronic venous congestion, arterial insufficiency or pressure sores. Some rare causes include rheumatoid arthritis, sickle cell anemia, hemolytic anemia, leukemia, acral melanoma or Marjolin's ulcer. Common features shared by each of the non-healing ulcers include prolonged or excessive inflammation, persistent infections, development of drug-resistant microbial biofilms, and the inability of dermal and/or epidermal cells to respond to reparative stimuli. A non-healing wound represents a significant clinical challenge and any lesion of this type should be biopsied in order to rule out a malignant cause of ulceration.

Onychomycosis represents the fungal infection of the nail that may associate the presence of longitudinal melanonychia when infected by dematiaceous fungi. Besides the change in nail colour, patients with onychomycosis may associate subungual hyperkeratosis, onychodystrophy or onycholysis. The most frequently involved fungus in the development of nail melanonychia due to melanin synthesis is *Trichophyton rubrum* [8]. When a fungal infection is suspected, the direct microscopic examination and fungal culture provide important clues although there are cases of inconclusive results when histology is required. Treatment is challenging, as these fungi are often not responsive to traditional antifungal therapy.

Key Points
- ALM is a common melanoma subtype found in dark-skinned and Asian populations.
- ALM tends to have a poor prognosis due to the advanced stage in the moment of presentation.
- The imprint histology may be a valuable diagnostic investigation in melanocytic lesions.
- Significant prognostic factors are represented by advanced age, the presence of ulceration, tumor thickness and tumor spread in the moment of diagnosis.
- Comprehensive skin examination, including the acral areas of the body, is of utmost importance in early diagnosis of ALM.

References

1. Desai A, Ugorji R, Khachemoune A. Acral melanoma foot lesions. Part 1: epidemiology, aetiology, and molecular pathology. Clin Exp Dermatol. 2017;42:845–8.
2. Reed RJ. New concepts in surgical pathology of the skin. New York: Wiley; 1976. p. 89–90.
3. Li H, Liu X. Acral lentiginous melanoma. Clin Oncol. 2018;3:1548.
4. Bristow IR, Acland K. Acral lentiginous melanoma of the foot and ankle: a case series and review of the literature. J Foot Ankle Res. 2008 Dec;1(1):11.
5. Teramoto Y, Keim U, Gesierich A, Schuler G, Fiedler E, Garbe C, et al. Acral lentiginous melanoma – a skin cancer with unfavourable prognostic features. A study of the German Central Malignant Melanoma Registry (CMMR) in 2050 patients. Br J Dermatol. 2018;178:443–51.

6. Phan A, Dalle S, Touzet S, Ronger-Savlé S, Balme B, Thomas L. Dermoscopic features of acral lentiginous melanoma in a large series of 110 cases in a white population. Br J Dermatol. 2010;162:765–71. https://doi.org/10.1111/j.1365-2133.2009.09594.x.
7. Radu O, Pantanowitz L. Kaposi sarcoma. Arch Pathol Lab Med. 2013 Feb;137(2):289–94.
8. Finch J, Arenas R, Baran R. Fungal melanonychia. J Am Acad Dermatol. 2012 May 1;66(5):830–41.

Chapter 26
Hypomelanotic Nodular Lesions in a 38-Year-Old Female

Alexandra-Irina Butacu, Ionela Manole, Sabina Zurac, and George-Sorin Tiplica

A 38-year-old, fair-skinned, blue-eyed female, from rural environment, with no significant medical personal or family history, presented for dermatological consultation with a single nodular lesion located on the dorsal-lateral side of the right upper arm (Fig. 26.1). Onset was 3 months prior, with a rapid evolution in terms of increasing in size. The patient reported pain as associated local symptomatology and frequent bleeding of the tumor after minor local trauma.

Fig. 26.1 A 38-year-old presented for consultation with a single nodular lesion located on the dorsal-lateral side of the right upper arm, with a 3 months evolution

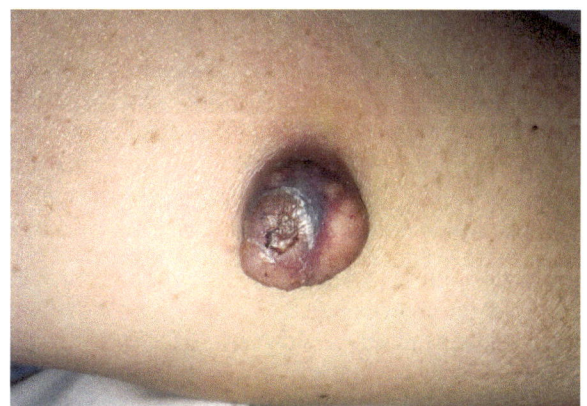

A.-I. Butacu · I. Manole · G.-S. Tiplica (✉)
2nd Department of Dermatology, Colentina Clinical Hospital, "Carol Davila" University of Medicine and Pharmacy, Bucharest, Romania

S. Zurac
Department of Pathology, Colentina Clinical Hospital, Bucharest, Romania

T. Lotti et al. (eds.), *Clinical Cases in Melanoma*,
Clinical Cases in Dermatology, https://doi.org/10.1007/978-3-030-50820-3_26

Fig. 26.2 Surgical
excision of the lesion was
performed and sectioning
of the lesion
macroscopically identified
scarce islands of
disorganized brown
pigment networks

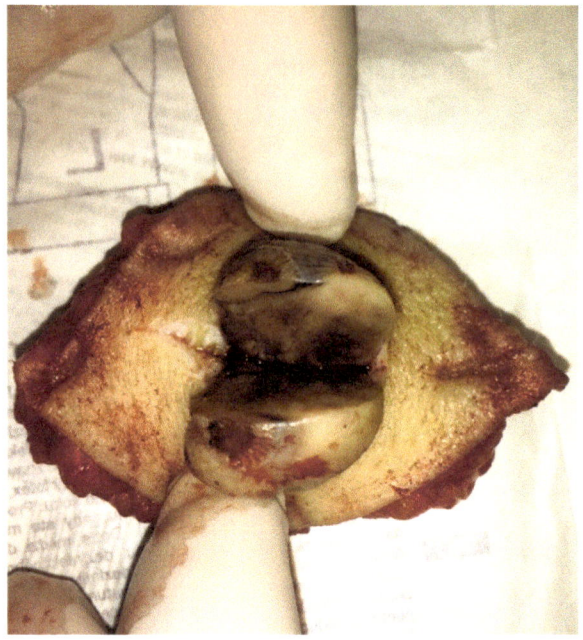

The physical examination revealed a ulcerated nodular lesion of 2.5 × 2 cm in diameter and 1.5 cm in height. The tumor was firm, circumscribed, covered by telangiectatic skin and with a apical small ulceration of 4 mm in diameter having fibrinoid deposit in its base. The lesion associated an erythematous-violaceous hue and an infiltrated base of 1cm in diameter.

Surgical excision and histopathological examination were performed under local anaesthesia (Fig. 26.2).

Based on the case description and the photograph, what is your diagnosis?

- Nodular melanoma
- Pyogenic granuloma
- Nodular basal cell carcinoma
- Merkel cell carcinoma.

Diagnosis

Hypomelanotic nodular melanoma, with hypodermal and lymphatic invasion, Breslow index of 20 mm, mitotic index of ten mitotic figures per mm^2, Clark level V (Fig. 26.3).

Fig. 26.3 The histopathological report described on Hematoxylin and eosin stain a melanocytic proliferation with micronodular architecture, composed of islands of polygonal cells with pleomorphic cyto-nuclear aspect and occasional deposits of melanic pigment; tumor thickness of 20 mm, a mitotic index of ten mitotic figures per mm² and hypodermal and lymphatic invasion

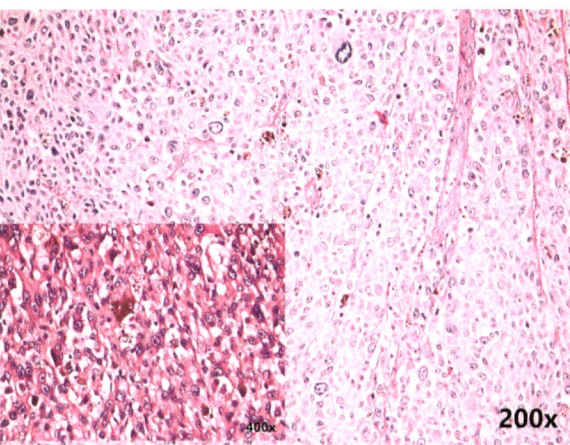

Discussion

Cutaneous melanoma represents 5% of malignant cutaneous tumors and is responsible for 75% of skin-cancer-related deaths. Four major subtypes are recognized, superficial spreading melanoma, nodular melanoma, lentigo malignant melanoma and acral lentiginous melanoma. Mean age of diagnosis is 52, which is significantly lower than mean age values of other frequent cancers, such as colo-rectal or prostate cancer. Nodular melanoma is the second most common form, following superficial spreading melanoma and represents 10–15% of all melanomas. Nodular melanoma usually arises de novo, on normally appearing skin and associates a uniformly distributed black-blue color. It is most frequently located on intermittently sun exposed areas, such as the trunk. Nodular melanoma is considered the most aggressive subtype, with a rapid evolution of weeks to months and an increased tumor thickness on the histopathological report [1].

Amelanotic/hypomelanotic melanomas represent 5% of nodular melanomas and 2–8% of all melanoma cases. Such lesions may lack characteristic clinical diagnosis criteria, for example asymmetry and disorganized peripheral pigmentation [2]. Therefore, clinical diagnosis is usually difficult due to the lack or decreased pigmentation and due to the diverse clinical presentations, often leading to delayed diagnosis or misdiagnosis, inappropriate treatment and a poor prognosis [3].

Pyogenic granuloma, also called lobular capillary hemangioma, may be confused with hypomelanotic nodular melanoma, due to its rapid evolution and vascularized clinical aspect. Pyogenic granulomas represent reactive proliferation of capillary blood vessels and usually appear as solitary red-purple papule or nodules, which bleed easily. Localization includes sites of previous local trauma, especially the extremities and the head and neck regions. Pyogenic granuloma is a benign lesion which may present spontaneous resolution or may require surgical treatment [4].

Nodular basal cell carcinoma is the most common form of basal cell carcinoma, the most frequent human cancer. Nodular basal cell carcinoma is a malignant proliferation of keratinocytes, which usually affects fair-skinned individuals between 60 and 80 years of age and is most frequently located on sun exposed areas such as the facial region. Local destructive potential is associated, with possible invasion of the subcutaneous tissues, muscle and bones, but risk of metastases is usually low [5]. Dermoscopy represents a useful tool in differentiating basal cell carcinomas from amelanotic/hypomelanotic melanomas based on the absence of a pigment network and the presence of specific features, such as arborizing vessels, large blue-grey ovoid nests, multiple blue-grey globules, leaf-like areas, spoke wheel areas and ulceration [6].

Merkel cell carcinoma, also called primary cutaneous neuroendocrine carcinoma, is a rare and aggressive tumor, frequently metastatic with an associated mortality of 30–40%. Its name is due to the ultrastructural and immune-phenotypical resemblance of neoplastic cells to sensory Merkel cells found in the skin. Most cases of Merkel cell carcinomas arise by the monoclonal integration of Merkel cell polyomavirus (MCPyV), while the remaining cases are associated with ultraviolet radiation exposure. Most cases affect the facial region of males after the age of 50 and present as single erythematous asymptomatic nodules which require differentiation from amelanotic/hypomelanotic melanomas [7].

Based on clinical and histopathological examinations, the diagnosis of hypomelanotic nodular melanoma was established. The patient was consecutively referred to the local Oncology Department.

Key Points
1. Nodular melanoma represents 10–15% of melanoma cases and is the most aggressive subtype.
2. Nodular melanoma usually arises on normally appearing skin, presents as a uniformly black-blue colored nodular lesion and is most frequently located on intermittently sun exposed areas.
3. Amelanotic/hypomelanotic melanomas usually present as nodular subtypes and represent 2–8% of all melanomas.
4. Amelanotic/hypomelanotic melanomas may lack characteristic clinical diagnosis criteria, such as asymmetry or disorganized peripheral pigmentation which often lead to delayed diagnosis or misdiagnosis, inappropriate treatment and a poor prognosis.
5. Amelanotic/hypomelanotic melanomas should be differentiated from pyogenic granulomas, nodular basal cell carcinomas, Merkel cell carcinomas.

References

1. Goldsmith L, Katz S, Gilchrest B, Paller A, Leffell D, Wolff K. Cutaneous melanoma. Fitzpatrick's dermatology in general medicine. 8th ed. New York: Mc Graw Hill Medical; 2012. p. 1416–45.
2. Moloney FJ, Menzies SW. Key points in the dermoscopic diagnosis of hypomelanotic melanoma and nodular melanoma. J Dermatol. 2011 Jan;38(1):10–5.
3. Steglich RB, Meotti CD, Ferreira MS, Lovatto L, Carvalho AV, Castro CG. Dermoscopic clues in the diagnosis of amelanotic and hypomelanotic malignant melanoma. An Bras Dermatol. 2012 Dec;87(6):920–3.
4. Moshe M, Levi A, Ad-El D, Ben-Amitai D, Mimouni D, Didkovsky E, et al. Malignant melanoma clinically mimicking pyogenic granuloma: comparison of clinical evaluation and histopathology. Melanoma Res. 2018 Aug 1;28(4):363–7.
5. Cameron MC, Lee E, Hibler BP, Barker CA, Mori S, Cordova M, et al. Basal cell carcinoma: Epidemiology; pathophysiology; clinical and histological subtypes; and disease associations. J Am Acad Dermatol. 2019 Feb 1;80(2):303–17.
6. Kato J, Horimoto K, Sato S, Minowa T, Uhara H. Dermoscopy of melanoma and non-melanoma skin cancers. Front Med. 2019;6:180.
7. Harms PW, Harms KL, Moore PS, DeCaprio JA, Nghiem P, Wong MK, et al. The biology and treatment of Merkel cell carcinoma: current understanding and research priorities. Nat Rev Clin Oncol. 2018 Dec;15(12):763–76.

Chapter 27
A 43-Year-Old Female With Nodular Lesion in the Hypogastric Region

Le Huu Doanh, Nguyen Van Thuong, and Michael Tirant

A 43-year-old female was admitted to surgery department with a painless tumor developing at hypogastric region for the past 4 years (Fig. 27.1). In the last 4 months, the lesion developed very quickly in size and became ulcerated and bleeding easily. She denied fatigue and weigh loss.

Fig. 27.1 A 43-year-old female presented complaining of big nodule at hypogastric region for the past 4 years

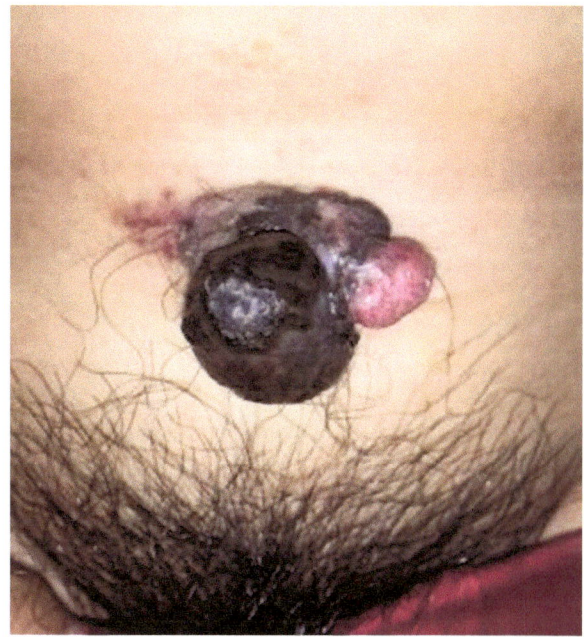

L. H. Doanh · N. Van Thuong · M. Tirant (✉)
Department of Dermatology, Hanoi Medical University, Hanoi, Vietnam
e-mail: drmichael@psoriasis.com.au

Base on the description and the photograph, what is your diagnosis?

1. Basal cell carcinoma
2. Melanoma
3. Squamous cell carcinoma
4. Cellular blue

She was administered several tests include biopsy with hematoxylin—eosin stain and the results was:

- Cell blood count was normal: RBC: 5.15 T/l, WBC: 6.41 G/l, PLT: 325 T/l
- Groin ultrasound reveals some well-defined lymph node in two sites with smooth clear margins and their sizes: 10.7 × 14.2 mm (right), 4.1 × 7.4 mm (left).
- PET CT showed bright spot at right groin and other organs were normal.
- Histopathology (Fig. 27.2): the epidermis seemed normal, the dermis had image of many atypical melanocytes which are smaller than normal and have large hyperchromatic nuclei, irregular nuclear shape and nuclear polymorphism, abnormal chromatin pattern, and prominent nucleoli. Marker S100, Melan A, Ki67, HMB45 stain were positive

An incision biopsy of the inguinal lymph node was administered with the results of chronic inflammation at the left inguinal lymph node but the right groin lymph node had many atypical melanocytes (Figs. 27.3 and 27.4).

Diagnosis

Metastatic nodular melanoma stage IIIC with T4bN1bM0.

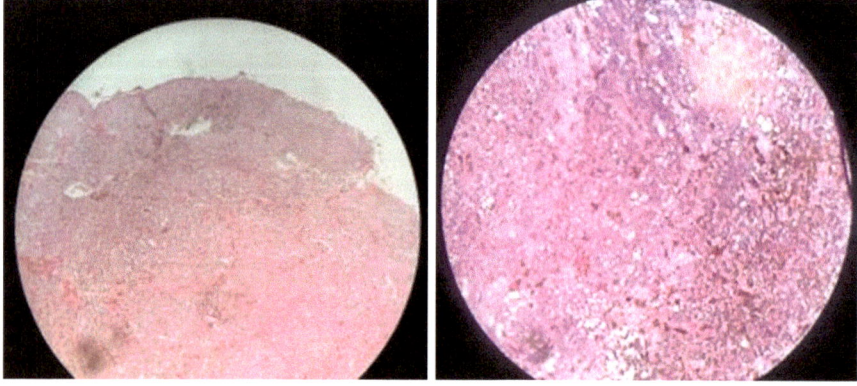

Fig. 27.2 Many atypical melanocytes, small, spindled, finely dusted with melanin, arise at the dermal-epidermal junction and invade the dermis. Pleomorphism, hyperchromatism, increased mitoses, and prominent nucleoli

Fig. 27.3 HMB45 stain
was positive

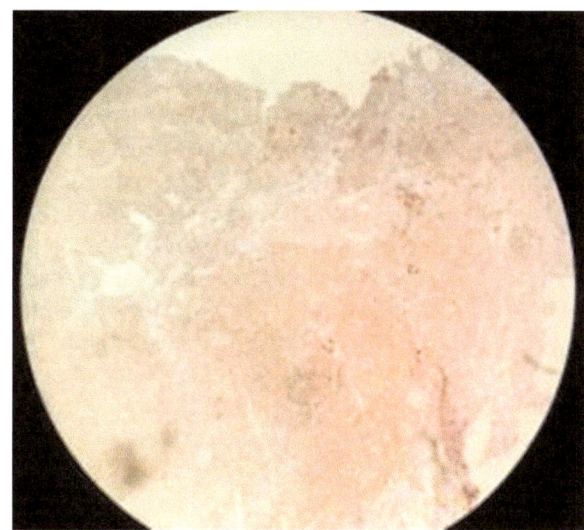

Fig. 27.4 Melan A stain
was positive

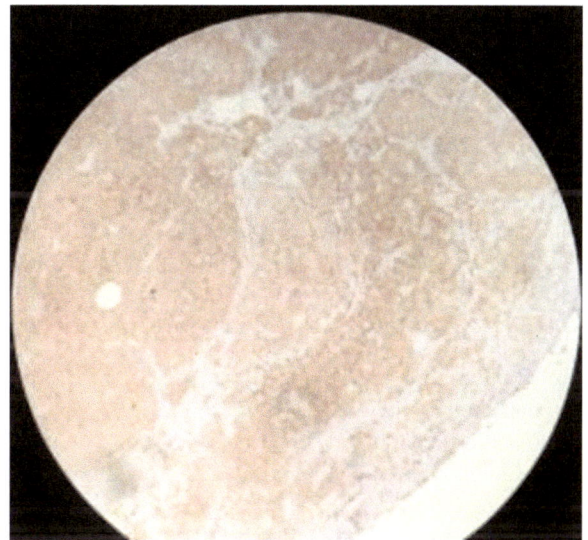

Discussion

Melanoma is a malignant tumor that arises from melanocytes, and accounts for only
4% of all skin cancer. Due to its metastatic potential, melanoma leads to more than
90% of skin cancer- related deaths.

Risk factors many be divided into three categories (1) genetic factors; (2) phenotypic manifestations of gene–environment interactions; and (3) environmental factors. The major high penetrative susceptibility gene locus associated with familial melanoma is CDKN2A and the strongest independent risk factors for the development of cutaneous melanoma are those that reflect a combination of genetic susceptibility and environmental exposure: melanocytic nevi, atypical melanocytic nevi, ephelides, and solar lentigines. The environmetal factors are UVB and UVA [1].

Nodular melanoma is the second most common type of cutaneous melanoma in fair-skinned individuals after superficial spreading melanoma and is diagnosed most frequently in patients in their sixth decade of life. It accounts for about 15% to 30% of all melanomas and can occur at any body site, but is most frequently seen on the trunk, head and neck. Nodular melanomas are observed more frequently in men than women. They usually present as a blue to black, but sometimes pink to red, nodule which may be ulcerated or bleeding and in some patients have developed rapidly over months. Nodular melanoma is believed to arise as a de novo vertical growth phase tumor without the pre-existing horizontal growth phase that characterizes the other histologic types. These melanomas tend to be diagnosed at a thicker, more advanced stage, with an associated poorer prognosis [1].

Histopathology remains the gold standard for melanoma diagnosis. In nodular melanoma, the tumor extends vertically in the dermis with a comparatively limited involvement of the overlying epidermis. About immune histochemical studies, melanocyte differentiation antigens, e.g. HMB45, tyrosinase, MART-1/Melan-A, S100 are useful for distinguishing cells of melanocytic lineage from other tumor types, for visualizing the full extent of tumor cells of a primary melanoma. HMB45 has high specificity for melanocytes and nevus cells, but its utility is limited by its heterogeneous staining pattern and more limited sensitivity than S100 [2].

Malignant melanomas was staged based on TNM classification. The prognosis and treatment was given based on stage. And 5-year survival of IIIC stage is only 40% [1].

Key Points
- Nodular melanoma is the second most common type of cutaneous melanoma in fair-skinned individuals.
- Nodular melanoma is believed to arise as a de novo vertical growth phase tumor without the pre-existing horizontal growth phase that characterizes the other histologic types.
- Nodular melanomas tend to be diagnosed at a thicker, more advanced stage, with an associated poorer prognosis.

References

1. Bolognia JL, editor. Dermatology: Expert consult, AJCC melanoma TNM classification – 2017. Edinburgh: Elsevier; 2017.
2. Rapini RP. Practical dermatopathology. Edinburgh: Elsevier; 2012.

Chapter 28
A 82 Year-Old Patient with Pigmented Lesion on the Sole

Nguyen Van Thuong, Le Huu Doanh, and Michael Tirant

An 82 year-old female presented to the hospital complaining of a gradually increasing size of macule on her left sole. The lesion was a flat hyperpigmented macule from the onset of two years ago. The patient reported no pain and no itching, thus she did not seek for any medical treatment. Recently, the lesion has had significant rise in size and she went to the hospital (Fig. 28.1).

Fig. 28.1 A pigmented lesion on her left sole with ill-defined border and irregular colour

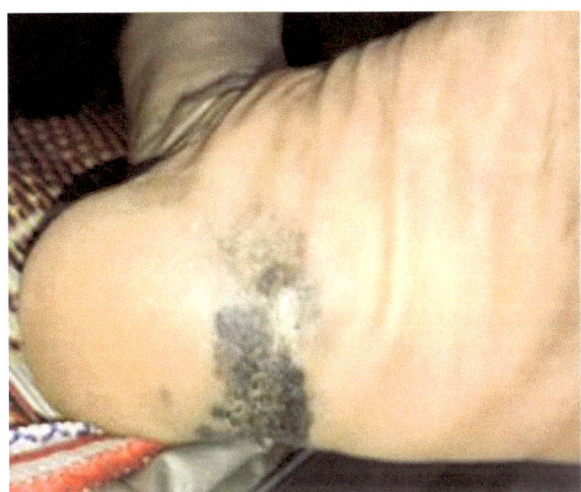

N. Van Thuong · L. H. Doanh · M. Tirant (✉)
Department of Dermatology, Hanoi Medical University, Hanoi, Vietnam
e-mail: drmichael@psoriasis.com.au

© The Editor(s) (if applicable) and The Author(s), under exclusive license to
Springer Nature Switzerland AG 2020
T. Lotti et al. (eds.), *Clinical Cases in Melanoma*,
Clinical Cases in Dermatology, https://doi.org/10.1007/978-3-030-50820-3_28

Fig. 28.2 Histopathology
revealed epidermis with
hyperplasia, Pagetoid cell
clusters in the epidermis;
dermis with inflammatory
reaction of monocytes

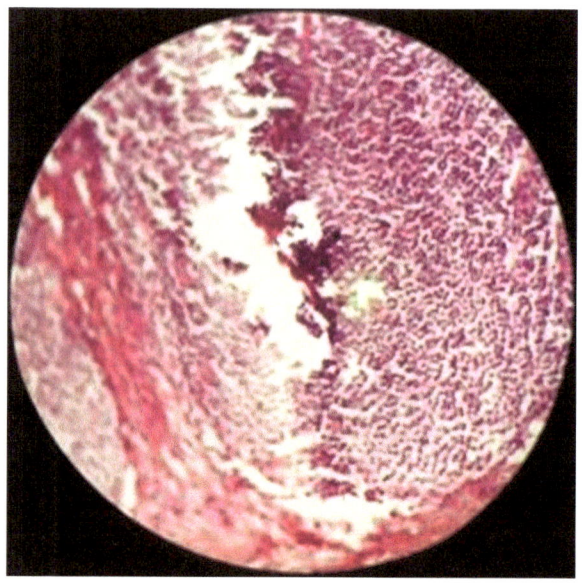

Based on the case description and the photograph, what is your diagnosis?

1. Atypical nevus
2. Basal cell carcinoma
3. Malignant melanoma

Biopsies for histopathology studies were obtained from her lesion and the result revealed a number of Pagetoid –like cells at the epidermis. Moreover, the basal membrane was not broken (Fig. 28.2):

Diagnosis

Melanoma.

Discussion

Melanoma is a potentially serious type of skin cancer, in which there is uncontrolled growth of melanocytes. Normal melanocytes reside in the basal layer of the epidermis and produce a protective melanin which protects cell skins by absorbing ultraviolet radiation. In various causes of melanoma, both genetic susceptibility and environmental risk factors, especially ultraviolet radiation, play a pivotal role through many mechanisms, including suppression the immune system of the skin, induction of melanocyte cell division and free radical production and damage of melanocyte DNA [1].

The disease generally affects the people aged from 40–50 years old. Melanoma often looks like black mole or nevi. Therefore, skin examination involves assessing the number lesions and distinguishing between of typical and atypical lesions. People can remember the abnormal features of melanoma by thinking of the letters A, B, C, D, and E [1]:

- Asymmetry—One half can look different than the other half.
- Border—It can have a jagged or uneven edge.
- Color—It can have different colors.
- Diameter—It is larger than 5mm
- Evolution—Its size, color, or shape can change over time.

Some melanoma lesions are itchy and tender. More advanced lesions may bleed easily or crust over.

Atypical nevi need to be distinguished with melanoma because it shares some same clinical features with melanoma and is considered as precursor lesions of melanoma. Unlike melanoma, atypical nevi is often found in trunk, especially the upper back in adults, the scalp and forehead in children. Although melanocytic nevi are harmless and do not need to be removed, it is not easy for an experienced dermatologist to tell whether a lesion is a nevus or a melanoma lesion, especially if there are atypical features. In those cases, dermoscopy could help. Besides, a suspicious or changing atypical nevus also should be removed by excision biopsy [2].

Another differential diagnosis for melanoma is basal cell carcinoma, especially nodular basal cell carcinoma because of its relatively rapid growth with bleeding as well as invasive nodular melanoma. Clinically, pigmented BCC shares the features of the corresponding histological subtype of its nonpigmented variants. It appears as a sharply demarcated nodule with a long- standing history of growth and often shows ulceration. Conversely, nodular melanoma usually starts as an expanding papule that increases in size quite rapidly. In addition, unlike melanoma, basal cell carcinoma happens in an older population (patients aged over 50 years-old). However both kinds of nodules, basal cell carcinoma and nodular melanoma cannot be distinguished by clinical examination alone. Dermoscopy and biopsy have to be required to be able to clarify the diagnosis [2, 3].

Key Points
- Melanoma is known as a malignant tumor that originates from melanocytes, and due to its metastatic potential, leads to >75% of skin cancer deaths.
- Atypical nevi and basal cell carcinoma are two main differential diagnoses for melanoma and sometimes, it is necessary to use biopsy for distinguishing.

References

1. Bolognia JL, Jorizzo JL, Schaffer JV. Neoplasms of the skin. In: Dermatology. 3rd ed. New York: Elsevier; 2012.
2. Goldsmith LA, Katz SI, Gilchrest BA. Fitzpatrick's dermatology in general medicine. 8th ed. New York: McGraw-Hill; 2012.
3. Morris-Jones R, Powell A-M, Benton E. 100 cases in dermatology. London: Hodder Arnold; 2011. p. 143–8.

Chapter 29
A Changing Pigmented Lesion on the Heel

Le Huu Doanh, Nguyen Van Thuong, and Michael Tirant

A 39-year-old man presented with a hyperpigmented macule on his left heel that progressively developed for 3 years. This lesion was non-itchy, painless and about 1 cm in diameter. He became hospitalized after that (Fig. 29.1).

Fig. 29.1 His lesion after a skin biopsy

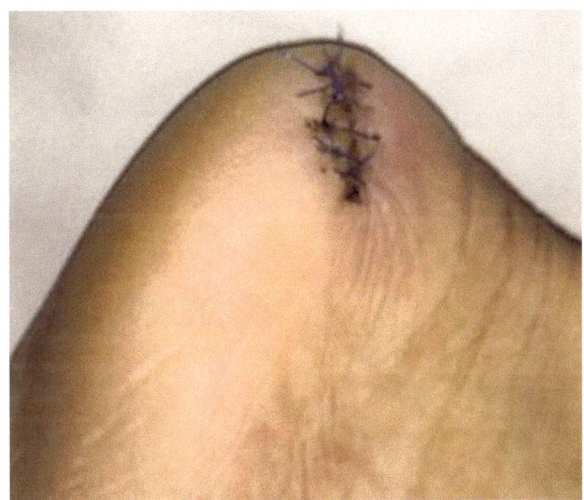

L. H. Doanh · N. Van Thuong · M. Tirant (✉)
Department of Dermatology, Hanoi Medical University, Hanoi, Vietnam
e-mail: drmichael@psoriasis.com.au

© The Editor(s) (if applicable) and The Author(s), under exclusive license to
Springer Nature Switzerland AG 2020
T. Lotti et al. (eds.), *Clinical Cases in Melanoma*,
Clinical Cases in Dermatology, https://doi.org/10.1007/978-3-030-50820-3_29

Based on the Case Description and the Photograph, What Is Your Diagnosis?

1. Malignant melanoma (MM)
2. Black heel (talon noire)
3. Benign acral melanocytic nevus
4. Post-inflammatory hyperpigmentation
5. Atypical mole
6. Pigmented basal cell carcinoma

A skin biopsy was performed and histopathology revealed melanoma with Breslow thickness 1.5 mm. Ultrasound revealed many inguinal lymph nodes with various sizes and unbroken structure (Fig. 29.2).

Diagnosis

Malignant melanoma.

Discussion

Malignant melanoma is a malignant skin tumor of melanocytes. It is the most aggressive type of skin cancer. Its incidence has doubled in the past decade. Malignant melanoma accounts for 5% of skin cancers, but incidence in the UK has

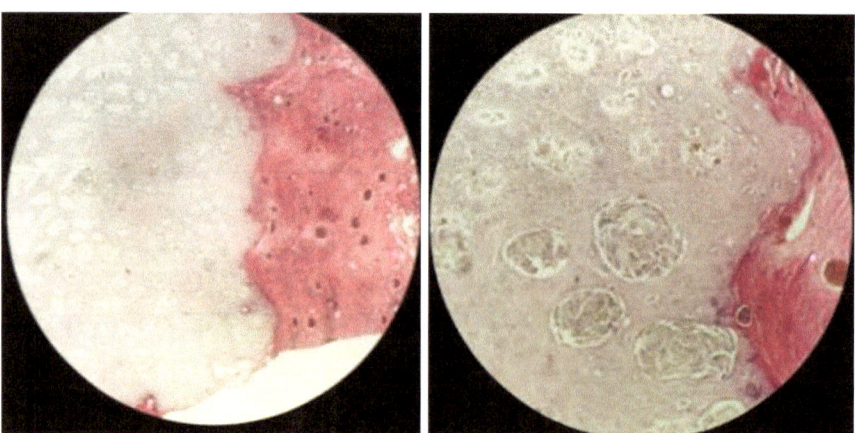

Fig. 29.2 Histopathology revealed epidermis with hyperkeratosis, pigmented clusters in stratum corneum and pategoid cell clusters; dermis with asymmetrical melanocyte hyperplasia, atypical melanocytes with enlarged melanocytic nuclei

Table 29.1 The main risk factors for developing the most common type of melanoma (superficial spreading melanoma)

Increasing age
Previous invasive melanoma or melanoma in situ
Previous basal or squamous cell carcinoma
Many melanocytic nevi (moles)
Multiple (>5) atypical nevi (large or histologically dysplastic moles)
A strong family history of melanoma with two or more first-degree relatives affected
White skin that burns easily
Parkinson disease

quadrupled since the 1970s (>13,300 new cases in 2013). Melanoma is commoner in men than women, and almost 1/3 occur in people aged <50 (melanoma is the commonest cancer in young adults aged 15–34 years old) [1]. Superficial spreading melanoma (SSM) is the commonest type in Caucasians. Approximately 30% of melanomas arise in a pre-existing nevus and the rest appear de novo. Malignant melanoma is more common in Fitzpatrick skin types I and II and has an increasing incidence closer to the equator. The etiology is complex, however it is known that genetic predisposition and ultraviolet light exposure (particularly intermittent sun-burning episodes) are likely to play a role (Table 29.1) [2].

A pigmented lesion that demonstrates significant change should be excised to exclude melanoma. The A-B-C-D-E rule of melanoma is a useful tool for determining if a lesion is suspicious:

- A—Asymmetrical shape.
- B—Border or Bleeding. The outline of a mole should be regular.
- C—Color. Benign nevi have a uniform color. Those nevi with differing pigment should be evaluated carefully.
- D—Diameter. Melanomas are usually >6 mm in diameter.
- E—Evolution: any change noted in a mole.

There are four main different variants of melanoma [3, 4]:

- Superficial spreading melanoma is the most common type and has a female preponderance. The lower leg is a common site. Clinically, the lesions are usually enlarging brown/black macules with irregular margins and varying degrees of pigmentation. Some lesions may show signs of regression (areas of paleness/whiteness within).
- Nodular melanoma is more common in men and is most frequently reported on the posterior trunk. Clinically, it appears as a pigmented papule or nodule that may ulcerate. During its horizontal phase of growth, the melanoma is normally flat, that is, superficial spreading melanoma. A nodular melanoma occurs as the vertical phase develops and the melanoma becomes clinically thickened and raised.
- Acral lentiginous melanomas occur on the palmar plantar regions and subungual sites. They are the most common form of melanoma in Fitzpatrick skin types

Table 29.2 Prognosis of malignant melanoma

American Joint Committee on Cancer (AJCC) stage	5-Year survival (overall >90%)
Stage 0 (melanoma in situ)	100%
Stage I (Breslow thickness <1 mm)	92–97%
Stage II	53–81%
Stage III	40–78%
Stage IV (metastatic disease)	15–20%

IV–VI. Acral melanomas may present as a pigmented macule or as a black area around the subungual skin and nail. The diagnosis is frequently delayed due to the skin sites affected and patients' lack of awareness, hence they often present late with a poor prognosis.

- Lentigo maligna melanoma is a melanoma that arises within a lentigo maligna (Table 29.2) [1, 5].

Key Points

- Malignant melanoma (MM) is the most aggressive type of skin cancer.
- It is more common in Fitzpatrick skin types I and II.
- Variants include superficial spreading, nodular, acral and lentigo maligna melanomas.

References

1. Griffiths CEM, Barker J, Bleiker T, et al. Melanoma. In: Rook's textbook of dermatology. 9th ed. Wiley Blackwell; 2016. p. 3973–94.
2. Bolognia JL, Jorizzo JL, Schaffer JV. Neoplasms of the skin. In: Dermatology, vol. 2. 3rd ed. Elsevier; 2012. p. 1885–915.
3. Kang S, Amagai M, Bruckner AL, et al. Melanoma. In: Fitzpatrick's dermatology, vol. 1. 9th ed. McGraw Hill; 2019. p. 1982–2016.
4. Burge S, Matin R, Wallis D. Tumours. In: Oxford handbook of medical dermatology. 2nd ed. Oxford University Press; 2016. p. 354–7.
5. Morris-Jones R, Powell A-M, Benton E. 100 cases in dermatology. Hodder Arnold; 2011. p. 143–8.

Chapter 30
A Dark Spot on the Right Sole

Le Huu Doanh, Nguyen Van Thuong, and Michael Tirant

A 54-year-old female presented with an irregular hyperpigmented lesion on her right sole that quickly progressively developed for 1 year. Her lesion was itchy, painless, and about 1.5 cm in diameter with a central ulceration that produced clear discharge (see Fig. 30.1). Before admitted, she went to private clinical and had unknown diagnosis and treatment but the lesion didn't improve.

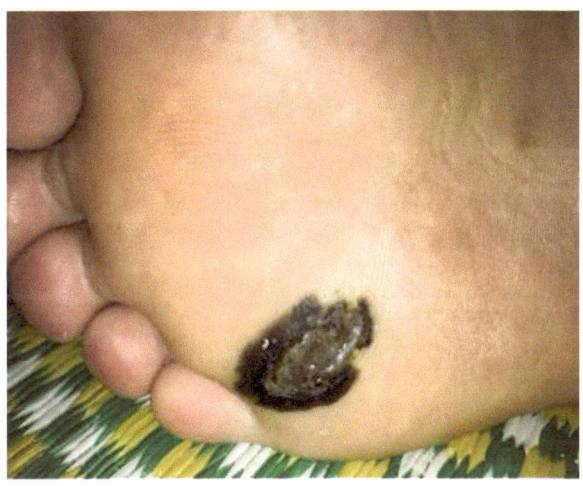

Fig. 30.1 Her lesion when she became hospitalized

L. H. Doanh · N. Van Thuong · M. Tirant (✉)
Department of Dermatology, Hanoi Medical University, Hanoi, Vietnam
e-mail: drmichael@psoriasis.com.au

Based on the Case Description and the Photograph, What Is Your Diagnosis?

1. Chronic trauma
2. Malignant melanoma
3. Melanocytic nevus

Dermoscopy suggested malignant melanoma (Fig. 30.2).

A skin biopsy was performed and histopathology revealed epidermis with pigmented clusters in stratum corneum and pategoid cell clusters; dermis with asymmetrical melanocyte hyperplasia, atypical melanocytes with enlarged and pleomorphic melanocytic nuclei and numerous melanin granules in cytoplasm; Breslow thickness was 1.5 mm; base on these findings, diagnosis of malignant melanoma was published.

Diagnosis

Acral lentiginous melanoma.

Discussion

Melanoma is a malignant tumor that arises from melanocytes and the most common form is cutaneous. Primary melanoma has four major subtypes, including superficial spreading melanoma, nodular melanoma, lentigo maligna melanoma and acral lentiginous melanoma. Besides, it has some subtypes that are not common such as

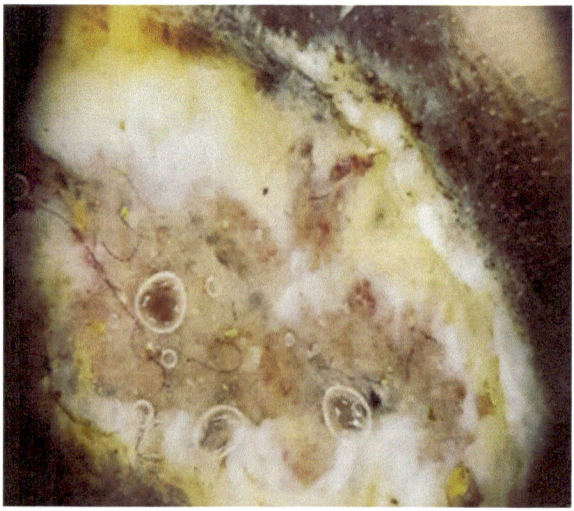

Fig. 30.2 Dermoscopy revealed a irregular asymmetric lesion with shiny white lines, polymorphous vessel hyperplasia, regression structures and blue-white veil sign

melanoma of the nail matrix and mucous melanoma [1, 2]. In this single case, the Vietnamese patient was diagnosed as acral lentiginous melanoma (ALM). Although ALM is a relatively rare form of melanoma and accounts for approximately 4–6% of all melanoma cases in white patients, it presents the most common expression of melanoma patterns in people with dark skins and Asians. Vietnam is a tropical country and many Vietnamese people are farmers with outdoor workplace. Therefore, the sun and ultraviolet light are known as factors in the causation of malignant melanoma. Other causes of its occurrence on soles must be considered [3]. The trauma of walking bare footed as is the customary with people in remote areas of the country could act as a trigger on genetic or familial factors or the presence of prepigmentation that could be premalignant lesions. Moreover, exposure to the agricultural chemicals also play a role of risk factors for ALM.

Normally, the diagnosis of melanoma may be delayed or missed particularly, especially with lesions on plantar. It may even be diagnosed with plantar warts, traumatic lesions and foreign body granulomas, pyogenic granuloma-like Kaposi sarcoma (PG-like KS) and hemangioma. Malignant melanoma is a serious disease with bad prognosis if diagnosis is missed or delayed. Its early detection and treatment give a better chance of survival for patients [2, 3].

American Academy of Dermatology (AAD) had a process after diagnosis [1]. It is helpful to treat and manage the patient. In this process often included these following steps (Fig. 30.3):

Earlier diagnosis of ALM is imperative so as physicians should maintain a high index of suspections and carry out comprehensive physical examinations for high-risk groups.

Fig. 30.3 Steps after diagnosis melanoma

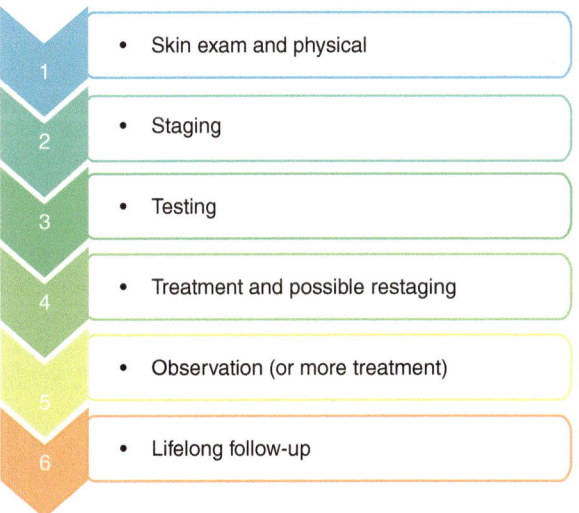

1 • Skin exam and physical

2 • Staging

3 • Testing

4 • Treatment and possible restaging

5 • Observation (or more treatment)

6 • Lifelong follow-up

Key Points

- Acral lentiginous melanoma is the most common melanoma in people with dark skins and Asians.
- The diagnosis of melanoma may be delayed especially with lesions on plantar.

References

1. Bichakjian CK, Halpern AC, et al. Guidelines of care for the management of primary cutaneous melanoma. J Am Acad Dermatol. 2011;65:1032–47.
2. Bolognia JL, Jorizzo JL, Schaffer JV. Neoplasms of the skin. In: Dermatology, vol. 2. 3rd ed. Elsevier; 2012. p. 1885–915.
3. Kang S, Amagai M, Bruckner AL, et al. Melanoma. In: Fitzpatrick's dermatology, vol. 1. 9th ed. McGraw Hill; 2019. p. 1982–2016.

Chapter 31
A Hyperpigmented Patch on the Sole

Nguyen Van Thuong, Le Huu Doanh, and Michael Tirant

A 62-year-old male presented to National Hospital of Dermatology and Vereneology with a 10-year history of a hyperpigmented patch on his right sole. 6 months before admitted, his lesion increased in size, and discharged. The lesion was painless, non-itchy, about 2 × 1.5 cm in size with irregular border (Fig. 31.1).

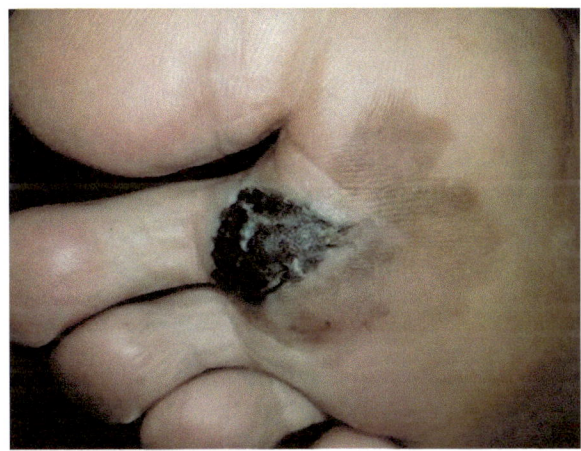

Fig. 31.1 A 62-year-old male presented with a hyperpigmented patch on his right sole

N. Van Thuong · L. H. Doanh · M. Tirant (✉)
Department of Dermatology, Hanoi Medical University, Hanoi, Vietnam
e-mail: drmichael@psoriasis.com.au

143

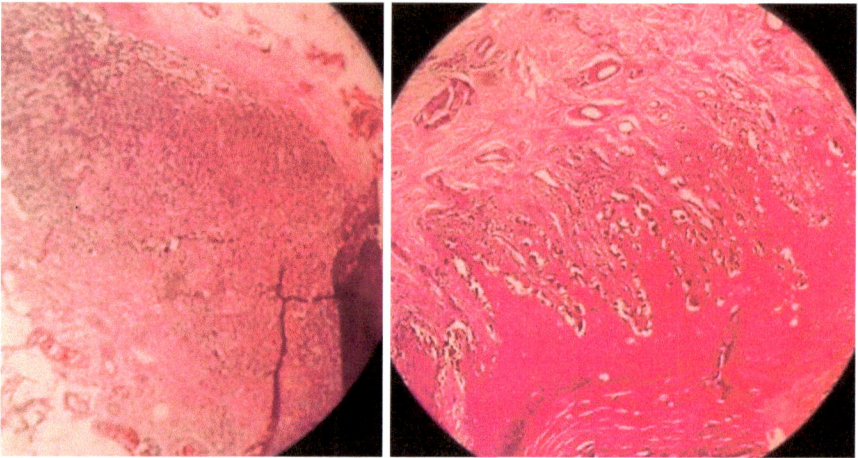

Fig. 31.2 Histopathology revealed epidermis with hyperkeratosis, pigmented clusters in stratum corneum and pategoid cell clusters; dermis with asymmetrical melanocyte hyperplasia, atypical melanocytes with enlarged melanocytic nuclei

Based on the Case Description and the Photograph, What Is Your Diagnosis?

1. Melanoma
2. Hyperpigmented basel cell carcinoma
3. Hyperpigmented Bowen's disease
4. Hyperpigmented serborrheic keratosis
5. Atypical nevus

Clinical findings suggested melanoma, so a skin biopsy was indicated. Histopathology revealed melanoma with Breslow thickness 1 mm (Fig. 31.2).

Diagnosis

Acral lentiginous melanoma.

Discussion

Melanoma is a potentially serious type of skin cancer, in which there is uncontrolled growth of melanocytes. The most frequent type is cutaneous melanoma but melanomas develop also at the mucosal, the uveal, or even the meningeal membrane.

Over the past several decades, incidence rates of cutaneous melanoma have increased significantly. It almostly affect in Caucasian population. The average age of people diagnosed with melanoma is 63. But melanoma is not uncommon even among those younger than 30. In fact, it's one of the most common cancers in young adults (especially young women).

Melanomas can form anywhere on the body, not only in areas that get a lot of sun. Although melanoma usually starts as a skin lesion, it can also rarely grow on mucous membranes such as the lips or genitals. Occasionally it occurs in other parts of the body such as the eye, brain, mouth or vagina.

The first sign of a melanoma is usually an unusual-looking freckle or mole. But with the atypical mole, we need to rule out melanoma by Glasgow 7-point checklist [1]:

Major features:

- Change in size
- Irregular shape
- Irregular color

Minor features:

- Diameter >7 mm
- Inflammation
- Oozing
- Change in sensation

With an atypical mole have these features, we need check by histopathology.

The best treatment for melanoma depends on the size and stage of cancer, patient's overall health, and personal preferences.

Treatment for early-stage melanomas usually includes surgery to remove the melanoma. A very thin melanoma may be removed entirely during the biopsy and require no further treatment. Otherwise, the surgeon will remove the cancer as well as a border of normal skin and a layer of tissue beneath the skin. For people with early-stage melanomas, this may be the only treatment needed.

If melanoma has spread beyond the skin, treatment options may include surgery to remove affected lymph nodes, chemotherapy, radiation therapy, biological therapy and targeted therapy.

In the last decades, completely new and effective treatment options for metastatic melanoma approved with immunotherapies such as the immune checkpoint blockade (anti-CTLA4, anti-PD-1 antibodies) and targeted therapies like BRAF/MEK inhibitors leading to a median overall survival of 2 years in stage IV melanoma and the chance for a long-term tumor control [2].

Key Points

- Melanoma is a potentially serious type of skin cancer.
- With an atypical mole, we need use Glasgow checklist. If it has some features of melanoma, we need indicate a skin biopsy to rule out melanoma.
- Melanoma is surgically curable if it's diagnosed at an early stage.

References

1. Bolognia JL, Jorizzo JL, Schaffer JV. Neoplasms of the skin. In: Dermatology, vol. 2. 3rd ed. Elsevier; 2012. p. 1885–915.
2. Kang S, Amagai M, Bruckner AL, et al. Melanoma. In: Fitzpatrick's dermatology, vol. 1. 9th ed. McGraw Hill; 2019. p. 1982–2016.

Chapter 32
A Middle-Aged Male with Hyperpigmented Lesion on the Heel

Nguyen Van Thuong, Le Huu Doanh, and Michael Tirant

A 54-year-old male farmer presented with a hyperpigmented macule on his right heel that developed for 3 years ago. His lesion was non-itchy, painless and increased in size rapidly and changed in color for 1 year. After that, he became hospitalized in National Hospital of Dermatology and Vereneology. Physical examination revealed not well-defined, irregular, 0.5-cm-diameter hyperpigmented plaque on the right heel (Fig. 32.1). No other lesions existed anywhere, and lymph nodes were not enlarged. The rest of medical history was normal and none of his family members had similar symptoms.

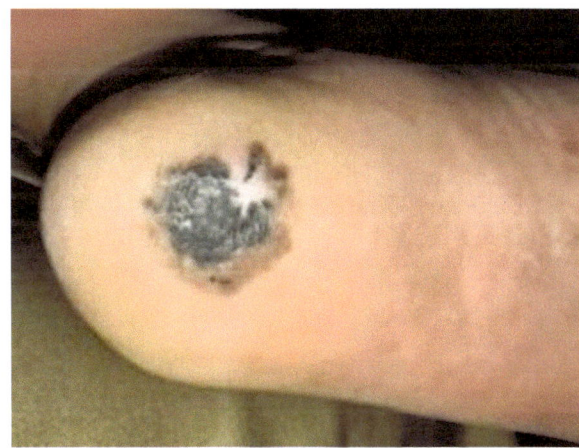

Fig. 32.1 The hyper-pigmented lesion with firm asymmetrical shape, irregular border, color variations, 2 cm in diameter, a little elevated surface in 54-year-old male patient

N. Van Thuong · L. H. Doanh · M. Tirant (✉)
Department of Dermatology, Hanoi Medical University, Hanoi, Vietnam
e-mail: drmichael@psoriasis.com.au

T. Lotti et al. (eds.), *Clinical Cases in Melanoma*,
Clinical Cases in Dermatology, https://doi.org/10.1007/978-3-030-50820-3_32

Based on the Case Description and the Photograph, What Is Your Diagnosis?

1. Malignant melanoma (MM)
2. Pigmented basal cell carcinoma
3. Benign acral melanocytic nevus
4. Post-inflammatory hyperpigmentation
5. Atypical mole
6. Pigmented Bowen disease
7. Seborrheic keratosis

Ultrasound revealed many inguinal lymph nodes with various sizes and unbroken structure.

All findings on dermoscopy suggested melanoma (Fig. 32.2).

A skin biopsy was performed by 2-mm excision margins; histopathology revealed melanoma and immunohistochemistry for S100 and HMB45 was positive (Fig. 32.3).

Diagnosis

Acral lentiginous melanoma in situ.

Discussion

Melanoma is the most serious form of skin cancer in which there is uncontrolled growth of melanocytes (pigment cells). Melanoma is sometimes called malignant melanoma. In the United States, it is the fifth most common cancer in men and

Fig. 32.2 Dermoscopy revealed hyperpigmented lesion in the form of stone mosaic, irregular edges, little scaly surface, regular brown-to-black dots surrounding lesion with vessel hyperplasia

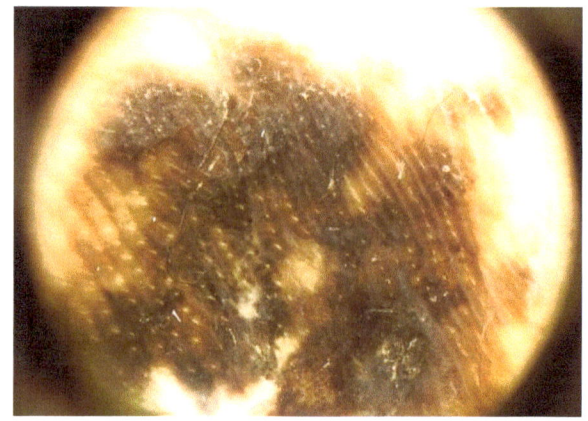

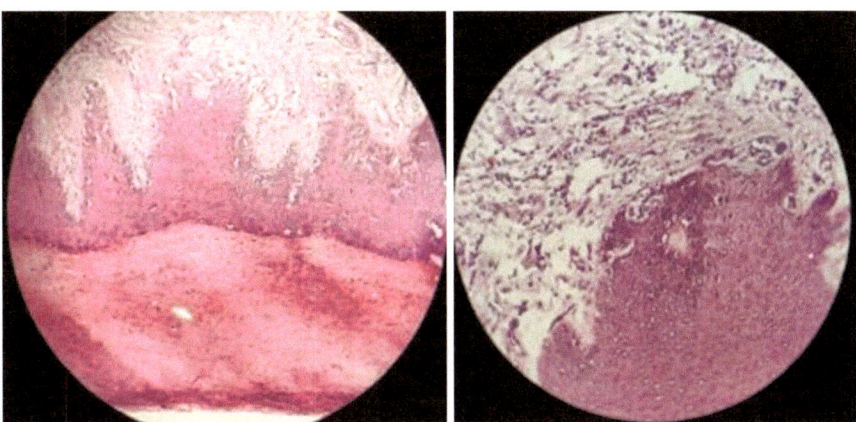

Fig. 32.3 Histopathology revealed atypical melanocytes that had larger size, large hyperchromatic nuclei, irregular nuclear shape and nuclear polymorphism, abnormal chromatin pattern, and prominent nucleoli and architectural disorders including asymmetry, poor circumscription, nests of melanocytes of various sizes and shapes in the lower epidermis and dermis. The epidermis penetrates the lichenic form of monon leukocyte

women; its incidence increases with age. Five-year survival rates for people with melanoma depend on the stage of the disease at the time of diagnosis. There are five stages (AJCC 8th edition melanoma TNM); stage 0 is in situ (intraepithelial) melanoma, stages I and II are localized invasive cutaneous disease, stage III is regional nodal disease, and stage IV is distant metastatic disease.

There are four major subtypes of invasive cutaneous melanoma including superficial spreading, nodular melanoma, lentigo maligna, and acral lentiginous [1].

The acral lentiginous subtype accounts for less than 5% of all melanomas. However, it is the most common type of melanoma among dark-skinned individuals (Fitzpatrick skin type IV and VI), who are at lower risk for more sun-related melanoma subtypes. Acral melanomas occur on the palmar plantar regions and subungual sites may present as a pigmented macule or as a black area around the subungual skin and nail. The diagnosis is frequently delayed due to the skin sites affected and patients' lack of awareness, hence they often present late with a poor prognosis. Acral lentiginous melanomas first appear as dark brown to black, irregularly pigmented macules or patches with raised areas, ulceration, bleeding, and/or larger diameter generally signifying deeper invasion in the dermis. Occasionally, acral melanoma can present as amelanotic or hypomelanotic lesions mimicking benign diseases, such as warts, calluses, tinea pedis, nonhealing ulcers, or ingrown toenails.

Hyperkeratotic cases of melanoma have often been mis-diagnosed. This case, was necessarily at a site of acute pressure regularly. So it appeared hyperkeratosis in lesion. Another reason for hyperkeratosis might be that our patient had tinea pedis. Coexistence of tylosis, clavus, human papilloma virus (HPV) infection, or other hyperkeratotic disorders may have an influence on keratinization of melanoma [2].

Table 32.1 Definitions of dermoscopic criteria for the 7-point checklist [1, 2]

Criterion	7-Point score
Major criteria	
Atypical pigment network	2
Blue-white veil	2
Atypical vascular pattern	2
Minor criteria	
Irregular streaks	1
Irregular pigmentation	1
Irregular dots/globules	1
Regression structures	1

Diagnosis total point ≥3

Table 32.2 Definitions of dermoscopic criteria for the 3-point checklist [3]

Criterion	Definition
Asymmetry	Asymmetrical distribution of colors and dermoscopic structures
Atypical network	Pigmented network with irregular holes and thick lines
Blue-white structures	Any type of blue and/or white color

Diagnosis of melanoma when all three criteria are suspected, suspected melanoma when lesions meet one criterion

Dermoscopy has been shown to be a useful and fairly inexpensive tool for melanoma detection in family practice. This technique can increase family physicians' confidence in their referral accuracy to dermatologists and can assist in decreasing unnecessary biopsies. Dermoscopy might be especially useful in examining patients at high risk of melanoma (Tables 32.1 and 32.2) [3].

Key Points

• Acral lentigo melanoma is the most common type of melanoma among dark-skinned individuals (Fitzpatrick skin type IV and VI)
• Dermoscopy has been shown to be a useful and fairly inexpensive tool for melanoma [3].

References

1. Davis LE, Shalin SC, Tackett AJ. Current state of melanoma diagnosis and treatment. Cancer Biol Ther. 2019;20(11):1366–79.

2. Kang S, Amagai M, Bruckner AL, et al. Melanoma. In: Fitzpatrick's dermatology, vol. 1. 9th ed. McGraw Hill; 2019. p. 1982–2016.
3. Kato J, Horimoto K, Sato S, Minowa T, Uhara H. Dermoscopy of melanoma and non-melanoma skin cancers. Front Med. 2019;6.

Chapter 33
A Pigmented Papular Lesion on the Heel

Nguyen Van Thuong, Le Huu Doanh, and Michael Tirant

A 71-year-old woman presented with an 18-month history of slow-extending pigmented lesion on her left heel. The patient described that the lesion initially appeared as a papule, then enlarged and recently has increased rapidly in size and has developed intermittently bleeding. Topical mupirocin prescribed by GP, had been ineffective so she was referred to the hospital.

Examination

She has an asymmetrical, papular, variably pigmented lesion, measuring 1.5–2 cm in diameter on her left heel. This has irregular border and several satellite pigmented lesions (Fig. 33.1).

Based on the case description and the photograph, what is your diagnosis?

1. Acral lentiginous melanoma
2. Tinea nigra
3. Verruca

Wide local excision was performed and histopathology showed an acral lentiginous melanoma with a Breslow depth of 3.5 mm.

Diagnosis

Acral lentiginous melanoma.

N. Van Thuong · L. H. Doanh · M. Tirant (✉)
Department of Dermatology, Hanoi Medical University, Hanoi, Vietnam
e-mail: drmichael@psoriasis.com.au

Fig. 33.1 An asymmetric
pigmented lesion,
1.5–2 cm in diameter with
several small satellite
lesions around on the
left heel

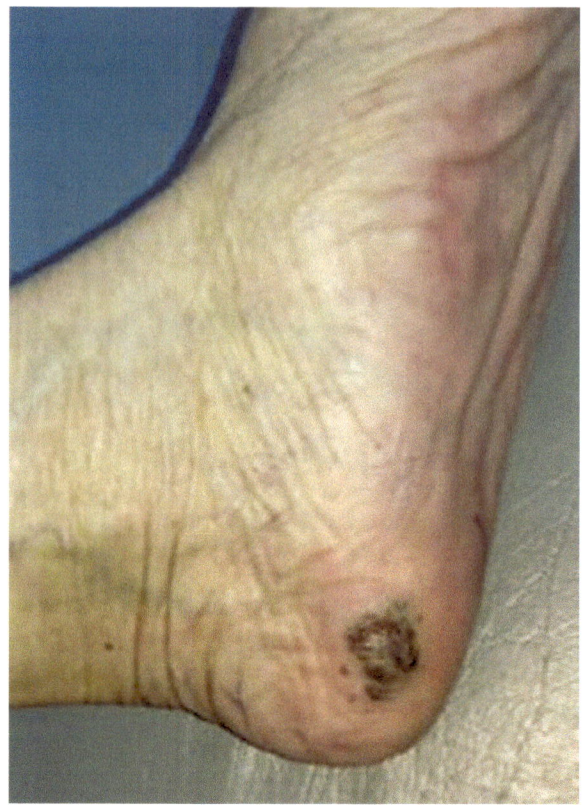

Discussion

This patient has a pigmented lesion on the heel that has changed in size, shape and color. The clinical appearance of this lesion should immediately raise the possibility of acral lentiginous melanoma.

A melanoma is a tumor produced by the malignant transformation of melanocytes. Melanoma is one of the most aggressive malignant skin tumors and its incidence has been increasing worldwide in recent decades. Annual incidence rates have increased among all populations, ranging from 3 to 7%, which results in a doubling every 10–20 years. About 75–80% of cutaneous melanomas seem to originate from normal skin. Therefore only 20–25% of melanomas are thought to develop in a cutaneous melanocytic nevus.

A pigmented lesion that demonstrates significant change should be excised to exclude melanoma. The ABCD rule of melanoma is a helpful tool for determining if a lesion is suspicious. However, many cases of seborrheic keratosis and atypical nevi fulfill the ABCD criteria whereas many melanomas do not [1].

A—Asymmetry

B—Border irregularity

C—Color variegation

D—Diameter > 6 mm

E—Evolution

Acral lentiginous melanomas (ALM) occur on the palmar plantar regions and sub-ungual sites. Among the 4 subtypes, ALM shows the highest incidence in Asian countries, whereas ALM comprises only 1% of all melanomas in white populations. They are the most common form of melanoma in Fitzpatrick skin types IV–VI. Acral lentiginous melanomas may present as a pigmented macule or as a black area around the subungual skin and nail. Early clinical diagnosis of ALM is essential, but early ALM lesions are often difficult to diagnose because the pigmentation of the lesions sometimes follows the skin marking of the palms and soles, resulting in an asymmetrical appearance and an irregular border in both ALM and benign melanocytic nevus. At later stages, ulceration or bleeding can occur, which should make diagnosis easier. To overcome this difficulty, dermoscopy was introduced, and determination of the patterns by this method is essential for accurate clinical diagnosis of ALM [1]. Pathological examination is still the gold standard for melanoma diagnosis, despite many attempt using molecular approaches to replace it. Any suspicious lesion of melanoma must be completely removed and sent for pathological examination (Fig. 33.2). The pathological analysis aims at confirming the malignancy and the melanocytic origin of the proliferation, but also to collect major prognostic information [2].

As with other types of melanoma, the standard therapy for primary ALM is wide local excision. The vertical level of the excision depends on the thickness of the tumor. As for the horizontal margins, wide local excision with 3- to 5-cm margins was previously recommended for the treatment of invasive melanoma. However,

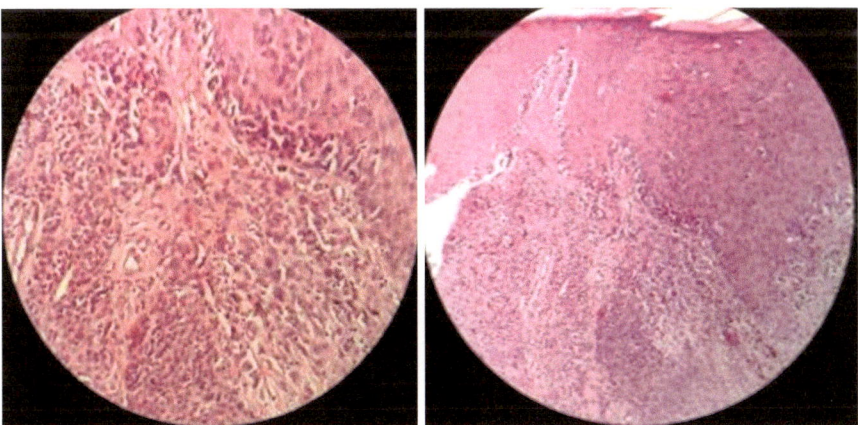

Fig. 33.2 Histopathology revealed proliferation of asymmetric melanocytes with poor circumscription; atypical melanocytes with enlarged and hyperchromatic nuclear invade the dermis

several studies have demonstrated no significant difference in overall survival or local recurrence rate between patients treated with narrow-margin excision and those treated with wide-margin excision. Balch et al. evaluated 2- versus 4-cm margins for melanoma of 1–4 mm in thickness and showed no significant difference in overall survival or local recurrence. In addition, Khayat et al. evaluated 2- versus 5-cm margins for melanoma of ≤2 mm in thickness in a randomized study and demonstrated no significant difference in the rate of recurrence or the 10-year overall survival rate. From these results, the current AJCC Guidelines recommend 1-, 1- to 2-, and 2-cm margins for invasive melanoma of ≤1, 1.01 to 2, and >2 mm in thickness, respectively [1].

After surgical excision, primary closure, skin grafting, secondary intention healing, and local and free flaps are performed with careful assessment of the functional and cosmetic aspects.

Tinea nigra is a superficial infection caused by dematiaceous fungi. The clinical skin lesion is characterized by well-circumscribed brown-black macule patches on the palms and soles. In Asia, such pigmentation on these areas can be suggestive of acral lentiginous melanoma. Potassium hydroxide test was positive for pigmented short hyphae. The lesion subsided following topical antifungal treatment without recurrence [3].

Palmar and plantar warts appear as thick, endophytic papules on the palms, soles, and lateral aspects of the hands and feet, with gently sloping sides and a central depression resembling an anthill. On the soles, these are painful from pressure when walking, due to their deep inward growth [4].

Key Points
- ALM is the most common form of melanoma in Fitzpatrick skin types IV–VI
- The ABCD rule of melanoma is a useful tool for determining if a lesion is suspicious
- Pathological examination is still the gold standard for melanoma diagnosis
- The standard therapy for primary ALM is wide local excision

References

1. Nakamura Y, Fujisawa Y. Diagnosis and management of acral lentiginous melanoma. In: Skin Cancer. T. Ito (ed) Current Treatment Opinions in Oncology 2018;14:42.
2. Grob JJ, Gaudy-Marqueste C. Rook's textbook of dermatology. Vol. Chapter 143. Oxford: Wiley-Blackwell; 2016.
3. Eksomtramage T, Aiempanakit K. Tinea nigra mimicking acral melanocytic nevi. IDCases. 2019;18:e00654.
4. Bolognia JL. Dermatology. 3rd ed. New York: Elsevier; 2012.

Chapter 34
A Pink, Dome-Shaped Nodule with Central Ulceration

Le Huu Doanh, Nguyen Van Thuong, and Michael Tirant

A 50-year-old female farmer presented with a bleeding ulcerative nodule on the right litle toe that developed for 3 months. She reported history of plantar wart on this site that was treated by four times of minor surgery. On cutaneous examination, there was a firm, 1 × 1.5 cm, dome-shaped, pink, nodule with a central ulceration covered by a yellow fine crust. Right inguinal lymph nodes were enlarged, firm, non-tender and ranged from 2 to 3 cm in diameter (Fig. 34.1).

Based on the case description and the photograph, what is your diagnosis?

1. Basal cell carcinoma
2. Intraepidermal squamous cell carcinoma
3. Amelanotic melanoma
4. Pyogenic granuloma
5. Keratoacanthoma

A skin biopsy was performed and histopathology revealed amelanotic melanoma with Breslow thickness 6.5 mm; immunohistochemistry for S100, Vimentin and HMB45 was positive (Fig. 34.2).

Diagnosis

Amelanotic melanoma.

L. H. Doanh · N. Van Thuong · M. Tirant (✉)
Department of Dermatology, Hanoi Medical University, Hanoi, Vietnam
e-mail: drmichael@psoriasis.com.au

T. Lotti et al. (eds.), *Clinical Cases in Melanoma*,
Clinical Cases in Dermatology, https://doi.org/10.1007/978-3-030-50820-3_34

Fig. 34.1 A 58-year-old
female presented with a
bleeding ulcerative nodule
on her right litle toe

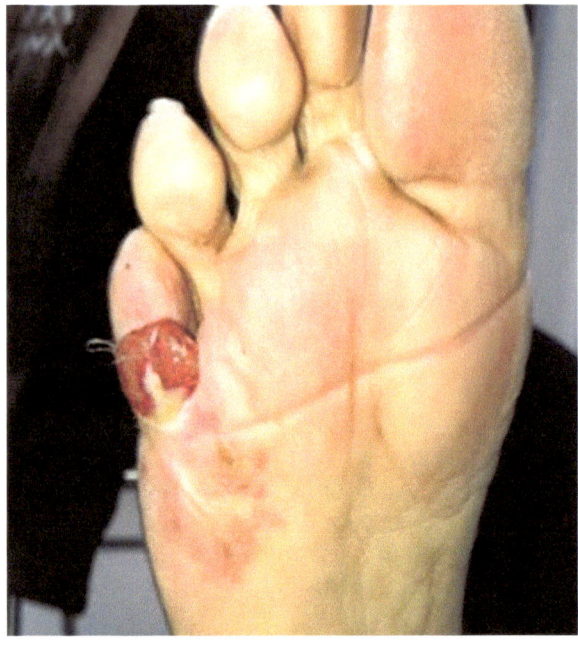

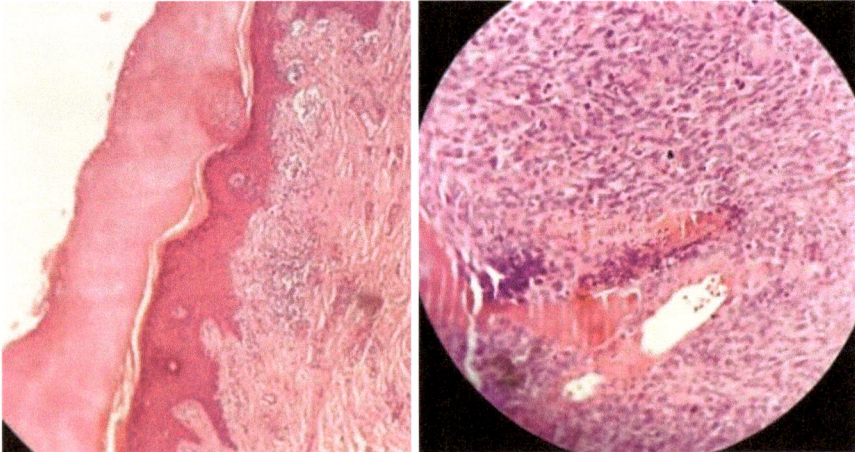

Fig. 34.2 Nests of atypical melanocytes at dermo-epidermal junction in papillary dermis

Discussion

Amelanotic melanoma (AM) is a subtype of cutaneous melanoma characterised by
little or no pigment on clinical examination. The term 'amelanotic' is often used to
indicate lesions that are only partially devoid of pigment while truly amelanotic

melanoma where lesions lack all pigment is rare. The incidence of AHM is appreciated to be 2–8% of all melanomas but the real incidence is difficult to estimate due to misdiagnosis.

Amelanotic melanomas may not display the clinical ABCDE criteria (Asymmetry, Border irregularity, Colour variation, large Diameter) that are classically used as melanoma warning signs. Patients and clinicians may not be alert to suspect non-pigmented lesions as melanoma and so amelanotic melanomas are often misdiagnosed. Expanding the ABCD warning signs to include the 3 R's (Red, Raised, Recent change) may help screen for amelanotic melanoma [1, 2].

There are four clinicopathologic variants of malignant melanoma including superficial spreading, lentigo maligna, nodular and acral lentiginous. AM can have any one of the above morphology but nodular is the most common variety. AM) may represent a primary melanoma, a recurrence of a previously pigmented melanoma, or a metastasis from pigmented primary melanoma [3, 4].

Dermoscopy, a non-invasive diagnostic method, improves the diagnostic accuracy of AHM. The characteristic dermoscopic features of amelanotic melanoma including Irregular pigmentation; irregular dots or globules) (in pigmented areas); polymorphous vascular patterns including milky-red areas, reticular depigmentation, dotted irregular vessels, linear irregular vessels, or the combination of dotted and linear irregular vessels; white lines [1].

Histopathology and immunohistochemistry are important tools for diagnosis of AM. In some cases, there is evidence of some pigment melanin on histopathology and immunohistochemistry, which includes S100 (positive for melanocytes) and HMB-45 (positive for premelanosomes).

Key Points
- Amelanotic melanomas account for around 2–8% of all melanomas.
- Amelanotic melanomas can lack classical features of other melanomas and tend to be red or skin colored and more symmetrical.
- Differential diagnosis includes basal cell or squamous cell carcinomas, pyogenic granulomas, and benign acral nail lesions.
- Histopathology and immunohistochemistry is essential tool for diagnosis of AM.

References

1. Pizzichetta MA, Talamini R, Stanganelli I, et al. Amelanotic/hypomelanotic melanoma: clinical and dermoscopic features. Br J Dermatol. 2004;150:1117–24.
2. McClain SB, Mayo KB, Shada AL, Smolkin MA, Patterson JW, Slinguff CL Jr. Amelanotic melanomas presenting as red skin lesions: a diagnostic challenge with potentially lethal consequences. Int J Dermatol. 2012;51:420–6.
3. Paek SC, Sober AJ, Hensin T, Martin C, Mihm MC, Johnson TM. Cutaneous melanoma. In: Wolff K, Goldsmith LA, Katz SI, Barbara AG, Paller AS, Lefffel DJ, editors. Fitzpatrick's dermatology in general medicine. 7th ed. New York: McGraw Hill; 2008. p. 1137–57.
4. Chatterjee M. Amelanotic malignant melanoma with multiple secondaries. Indian J Dermatol Venereol Leprol. 2006;72:252.

Chapter 35
An Elderly Male with Black Macule on Heel

Le Huu Doanh, Nguyen Van Thuong, and Michael Tirant

A 66-year-old male patient presented to the hospital with a gradually changing size of macule on the lateral side of heel (Fig. 35.1). The onset was 5 years ago with a flat hyperpigmentation macule. The lesion were painless and non-itchy so he did not seek for any treatment. Over the last 2 years, the lesion have gradually increased in size and appeared rough surface, therefore, he went to hospital.

Based on the case description and the photograph, what is your diagnosis?

1. Malignant melanoma
2. Atypical nevi
3. Basal cell carcinoma
4. Squamous cell carcinoma

This patient went to National Hospital of Dermatology and Venereology Vietnam and was given biopsy test twice but the results did not meet all the criteria of melanoma. Therefore, he returned his home and continued to monitor the progress of the disease. This time of admission, the clinical examination showed:

- A 3 × 1.5 cm vasodilatory hyperpigmented lesion, irregular border, rough surface with dark crust
- The satellite lesion is 1 cm in size
- Bilateral inguinal lymph nodes about 2 cm in diameter are palpable, mobile.

L. H. Doanh · N. Van Thuong · M. Tirant (✉)
Department of Dermatology, Hanoi Medical University, Hanoi, Vietnam
e-mail: drmichael@psoriasis.com.au

© The Editor(s) (if applicable) and The Author(s), under exclusive license to
Springer Nature Switzerland AG 2020
T. Lotti et al. (eds.), *Clinical Cases in Melanoma*,
Clinical Cases in Dermatology, https://doi.org/10.1007/978-3-030-50820-3_35

Fig. 35.1 An 66-year-old male presented complaining of a gradually changing size and rough surface of macule on the outside of the left heel with the characteristics: *A* asymmetric, *B* border irregularity, *C* color variation, *D* diameter over 6 mm, *E* evolution over time

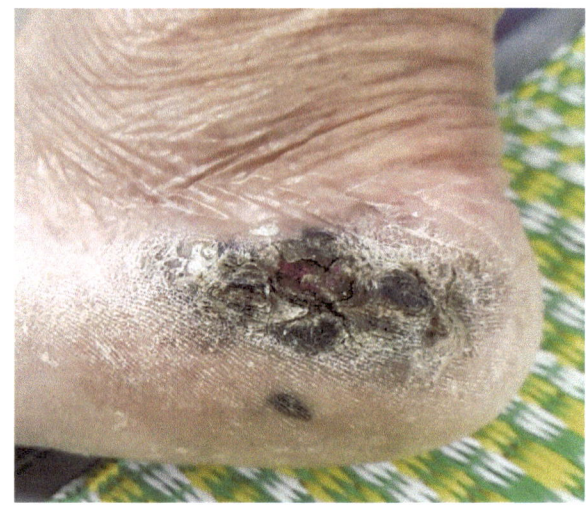

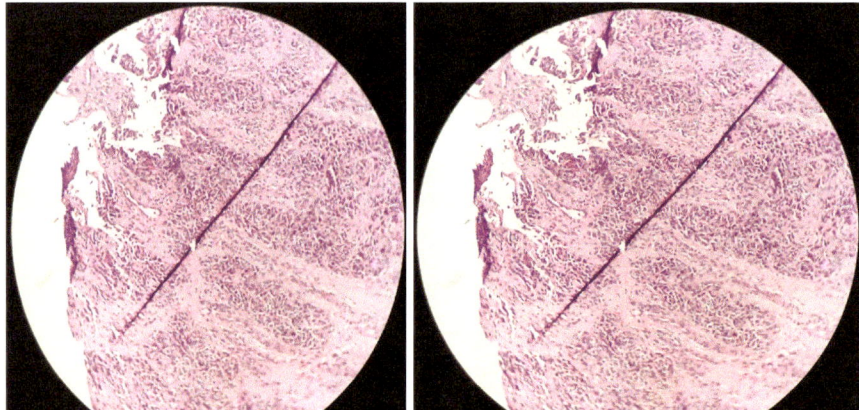

Fig. 35.2 The results of Hematoxylin Eosin staining were consistent with Melanoma, Breslow 2 mm

His entire lesion was removed and sent to the histopathology department. The results of Hematoxylin-Eosin staining were consistent with Melanoma, Breslow 2 mm (Fig. 35.2) with the characteristics:

- The epidermis is hyperkeratosis with pigmented clusters in stratum corneum and pagetoid cell clusters.
- The dermis is asymmetrical melanocyte hyperplasia, irregular border. Atypical melanocyte cells with small size, enlarged melanocytic nuclei, catch alkaline color, invasive to the dermis.

In this case, the patient was assigned to take PET-CT scan, which determined the patient had melanoma with bilateral inguinal lymph node metastasis.

Diagnosis

Malignant melanoma.

Discussion

Melanoma represents a malignant tumor which arises from melanocytes which are derived from the neural crest. This condition usually occurs on the skin, however, it can appear in other locations where neural crest cells migrate, such as gastrointestinal tract and brain. The melanocytes, which reside in the skin and produce a protective melanin, are contained within the basal layer of the epidermis. Although the explanation about causes of melanoma is unknown well, it may be related to both genetic susceptibility and environmental risk factors, especially ultraviolet radiation through many mechanisms, including suppression the immune system of the skin, induction of melanocyte cell division, free radical production and damage of melanocyte DNA.

Melanoma usually occurs in adults, about 40–60 years old. Melanoma is described as:

- In situ, if a tumor is confined to the epidermis
- Invasive, if a tumor has spread into the dermis
- Metastatic, if a tumor has spread to other tissues.

The characteristics of melanoma are commonly known by the ABCDE rule as following:

- A—Asymmetry
- B—Irregular border
- C—Color variations, especially red, white, and blue tones in a brown or black lesion
- D—Diameter greater than 6 mm
- E—Elevated surface

Also, melanomas may itch, bleed, ulcerate, or develop satellites. Patients who present with metastatic disease or with primary sites other than the skin have signs and symptoms related to the affected organ system(s).

It is also important to examine all lymph node groups.

Metastatic workup should be considered in patients that have melanomas greater than 4 mm, ulceration, satellite lesions, or any lesion that is recurrent. Metastatic workup is required for patients with regional disease:

- CT chest, abdomen, and pelvis with IV contrast
- MRI of the brain
- PET CT has been shown to be highly sensitive [1–3].

Key Points
- Melanoma represents a tumor which arises from melanocytes which mainly occurs on the skin.
- Melanoma is usually diagnosed in adults, about 40–60 years old.
- Histopathology is the gold standard in diagnosis.

References

1. Ott PA. Intralesional cancer immunotherapies. Hematol Oncol Clin North Am. 2019;33(2):249–60.
2. Tarhini A, Atzinger C, Gupte-Singh K, Johnson C, Macahilig C, Rao S. Treatment patterns and outcomes for patients with unresectable stage III and metastatic melanoma in the USA. J Comp Eff Res. 2019;8(7):461–73.
3. El Sharouni MA, Witkamp AJ, Sigurdsson V, van Diest PJ. Trends in sentinel lymph node biopsy enactment for cutaneous melanoma. Ann Surg Oncol. 2019;26(5):1494–502.

Chapter 36
Focal and Acral

Nguyen Van Thuong, Le Huu Doanh, and Michael Tirant

A 54-years-old female patient admitted to the hospital with a mild painful hyperpigmentation. The lesion began 3 year ago, initially with some hyperpigmented macules near her right heel. She scratched the lesion by a needle, then it spread widely. The patient was treated with laser therapy 2 years ago, but it was not completely cured. In this year, she continued scratching the hyperpigmented lesion nearby, then it spread more, bleed and oozed, appeared ulceration and dark crust. Her past medical history was normal (Fig. 36.1).

Base on the case description and the photograph, what is your diagnosis?

1. Hematoma
2. Pigmented basal cell carcinoma
3. Acral melanoma
4. Palmoplantar nevus
5. Plantar wart

On examination, she had a 2 × 3 cm dark pigmented plaque, irregular border on the right heel. The lesion had vasodilation and oozing. There is also variable pigmentation on the region of 5 × 6 cm around. After hospitalization, patient had biopsies of lesion at 5 sites. Biopsy results showed that 2 out of 5 sites are suspected of Melanoma, with Breslow depth of 2 mm and 2.1 mm, respectively. Immunofluorescence-based immunohistochemistry biopsies showed positive of S100 protein and HMB-45 (Fig. 36.2).

N. Van Thuong · L. H. Doanh · M. Tirant (✉)
Department of Dermatology, Hanoi Medical University, Hanoi, Vietnam
e-mail: drmichael@psoriasis.com.au

Fig. 36.1 A hyperpigmented lesion on the right heel of a 54-year-old female

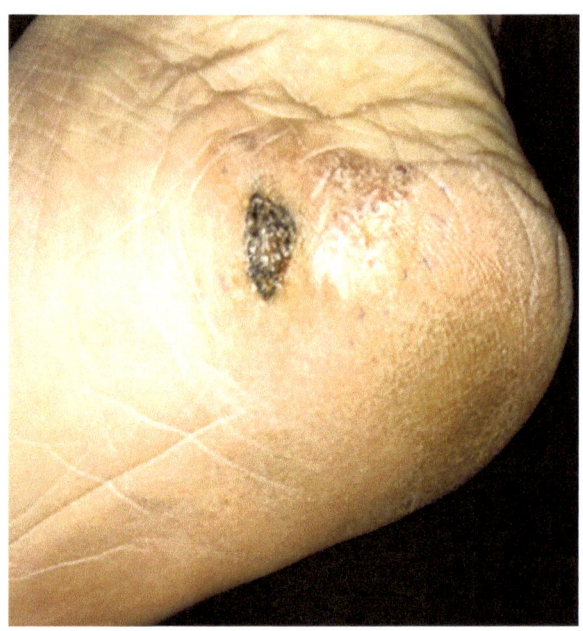

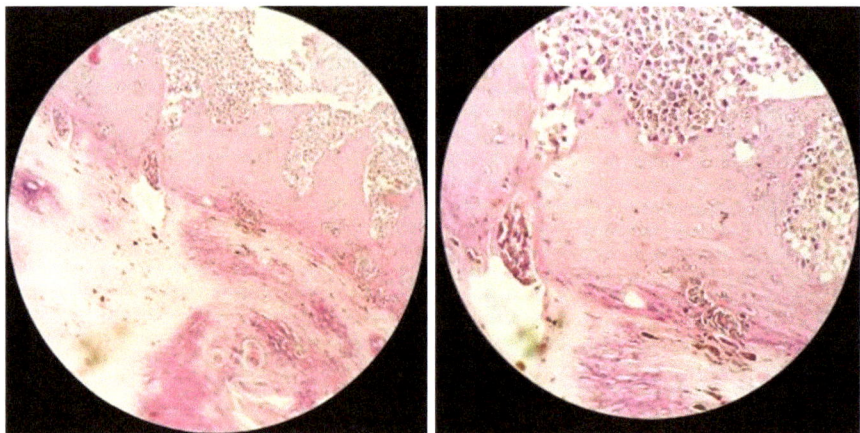

Fig. 36.2 Pathological pictures of biopsy piece number 2 (with Breslow depth 2.1 mm) at 20× and 40× magnification.

Diagnosis

Acral melanoma.

Discussion

Localized or '*focal*' hyperpigmentation may be due to melanin, hemosiderin or external-derived pigment. Focal hyperpigmentation is most often post-inflammatory, occurring after injury or other causes of inflammation (e.g., acne, lupus). Focal linear hyperpigmentation is commonly due to phytophotodermatitis, which is a phototoxic reaction that results from ultraviolet light. Focal hyperpigmentation can also result from neoplastic processes (e.g., lentigines, melanoma), melasma, freckles, or even café-au-lait macules. '*Acral*', pertaining to peripheral body parts, means the distal portions of the limbs (hand, foot) and the head (ears, nose). There are various causes of acral hyperpigmentation varying from genetic to acquired, benign to malignant, autoimmune to infectious, drug-induced, nutritional deficiencies, post-inflammatory, and even exogenous reasons [1].

There are many approach to focal hyperpigmentation according to the location of the lesion, for example the face, lips, extremities, trunk. Acral focal hyperpigmentation has many causes; but a focal lesion, as shown in the photograph, which presents in middle-aged patient with gradually spreading, no history of injury, does not respond to laser therapy as the patient we are discussing about, a malignant lesion cannot be ignored and a biopsy is needed.

Patient's histopathology and immunohistochemistry confirmed the diagnosis of Acral Melanoma. Melanoma is a malignant tumor that derived from melanocytes, mainly in the skin. Melanoma is a malignant disease that accounts for a small percentage of cancers in general and skin cancers so, but it's degree of malignancy and mortality are not that 'small'. The incidence rate of Melanoma has increased over the years, and Melanoma is also one of the most common cancers in young adults. Melanoma has four major subtypes, but it can also manifest very diverse based on clinical features and histologic findings. Acral melanoma (AM) is one of four subtypes, besides Superficial Spreading Melanoma (SSM), Nodular Melanoma and Lentigo Malignant Melanoma (LMM).

Acral melanoma is a rare subtype of cutaneous malignant Melanoma, AM only accounts for 2–3% of all malignant Melanoma, however, the palms, soles or in and around the nail apparatus regions are the most predominant sites of malignant melanoma in Asians, Africans and Latin American descent, who does not typically develop sun-related melanomas. AM is diagnosed more often in older patients, and compared with other subtypes of Melanoma, is associated with a lower incidence of familial Melanoma and lower number of common and atypical nevi. There is also a delay in the diagnosis of AM, often misdiagnosed as a plantar wart or hematoma, leading to a more advanced lesion upon diagnosis associated with poorer outcomes. Unlike most subtypes of Melanoma, AM is not thought to be associated with sun exposure. Some authors believe that moles in an easily traumatic region, such as the hands, feet, or shaving areas, are at high risk of turning into cancer and recommend early removal [1, 2].

The precise pathogenesis of AM continues to be investigated, but genetic alterations and trauma have been implicated. *CDKN2A, BRAF, RAS* and *PTEN* are all genes that have been well established as playing a major role in Melanoma, but their role in the AM subtype has only recently been investigated. AM is a genetically distinct subtype of melanoma and clearly differs from the other types of cutaneous melanoma, it harbors more and different genetic changes than the other types. *KIT* mutations and/or amplifications are more commonly identified in Melanomas located on acral and mucosal surfaces than on intermittently sun-exposed areas. *KIT* is an oncogene that encodes a transmembrane tyrosine kinase receptor, which leads to activation of the mitogen-activated protein kinase (MAPK) signaling transduction pathway, similar to that seen with *BRAF* mutations. A study by Torres-Cabala et al., the frequency of activating *KIT* gene mutations in AM was 15%. *KIT* gene mutations in exons 11, 13 and 17 were observed, and the L576P mutation in exon 11 was the most frequently detected. KIT gene mutation also opens the direction of targeted therapy, with early evidence that tyrosine kinase inhibitors (such as Imatinib) can be used for treatment. On the other hand, amplifications of the *CCND1* and *CKD4* genes have also been identified in AM (two critical G1 cell-cycle proteins and two genes that are transcriptionally induced by activated MAPK signaling), which leads to dysregulation of the cell cycle at the G1–S checkpoint [3].

Clinically, AM may develop in the hands, feet or subungual region, especially in the heel area with accounting for over 50% of Melanoma in the feet. Differential diagnosis of Acral melanoma (including subungual melanoma) is some hyperpigmented conditions that often appear in the acral region, such as Plantar wart, Palmoplantar nevus, Longitudinal melanonychia, Onychomycosis, Pyogenic granuloma and importantly Hematoma. Because of the delay in the diagnosis of AM (with a rate of >30%, misdiagnosis of AM appears to be more common than for other subtypes), if there is clinical suspicion of AM, an excisional biopsy is warranted. Diagnosis of AM can be made based on confirmation of the characteristic histopathology. In some cases, if the histopathological results are suspected or uncertain, some immunohistochemical markers should be used to confirm diagnosis, in which, S-100 is the most sensitive marker for melanocytic lesions, besides HMB-45, MART-1/Melan-A, Tyrosinase, and MITF. At the advanced stages, AM is easier for diagnosis, Saida et al. reported that acquired, large (>7 mm diameter), flat, heavily pigmented lesions are almost always melanoma, but then the prognosis is worse [4, 5].

Key Points
- Acral melanoma, one of four main Melanoma subtypes, is the most common types of Melanoma in Asians.
- AM presents in the palms, soles or in and around the nail apparatus regions, and is not associated with sun-exposure.
- Differs from the other types, *KIT* gene mutations are more commonly identified in acral type of Melanoma.
- AM often misdiagnoses as a plantar wart or hematoma. Early excisional biopsy is required to confirm diagnosis and increase patient's outcome.
- S-100 is the most sensitive immunohistochemical marker for melanocytic lesions.

References

1. Desai A, Ugorji R, Khachemoune A. Acral melanoma foot lesions. Part 2: clinical presentation, diagnosis, and management. Clin Exp Dermatol. 2017;43(2):117–23.
2. Saida T. Malignant melanoma on the sole: how to detect the early lesions efficiently. Pigment Cell Res. 2000;13(Suppl):135–9.
3. Torres-Cabala CA, Wang WL, Trent J, et al. Correlation between KIT expression and KIT mutation in melanoma: a study of 173 cases with emphasis on the acral-lentiginous/mucosal type. Mod Pathol. 2009;22:1446–56.
4. Bailey EC, Sober AJ, Tsao H, et al. Cutaneous melanoma. In: Fitzpatrick's dermatology in general medicine, vol. I. 8th ed. New York: The McGraw-Hill; 2012. p. 1416–44.
5. Garbe C, Bauer J. Melanoma. In: Bolognia JL, Jorizzo JL, Schaffer JV, editors. Dermatology, vol. II. 3rd ed. London: Elsevier Saunders; 2012. p. 1885–94.

Chapter 37
Middle-Aged Man with Hypopigmented Macules

L. Trane, R. Colucci, and S. Moretti

A 60-year-old caucasian man experienced an appearance of hypopigmented macules on his face, trunk, hands and legs. He reffered that he had been suffering from this condition for the last 3 years. The outset was gradual with a fast expansion.

The medical history of his family -his mother- was suggestive for melanoma and he had been suffering from autoimmune hypothyroidism for 30 years -treated with levothyroxine-, hypertension and hypercholesterolaemia. Furthermore, 4 years earlier he had an excision of melanoma of his abdomen (superficial spreading melanoma 0.4 mm Breslow thickness, 1 mitosis, with a marked regression). Sentinel lymph node biopsy was positive.

Based on the Case Description and the Photographs, What Is Your Diagnosis?

1. Melanoma-associated leucoderma
2. Vitiligo
3. Post-inflammatory hypopigmentation
4. Pityriasis Alba

On Wood's lamp examination the hypopigmented area involved most of the trunk, back, legs and face; without a marked fluorescence. The patient was treated with local low-potency corticosteroids, without a clinically relevant benefit (Figs. 37.1, 37.2 and 37.3).

L. Trane (✉) · R. Colucci · S. Moretti
Section of Dermatology – Department of Dermatological Sciences, University of Florence, Florence, Italy
e-mail: silvia.moretti@unifi.it

T. Lotti et al. (eds.), *Clinical Cases in Melanoma*,
Clinical Cases in Dermatology, https://doi.org/10.1007/978-3-030-50820-3_37

Fig. 37.1 On Wood's
Lamp examination flecked
hypopigmented coalescent
macules widely spread
on the back of a 60-year-
old caucasian man

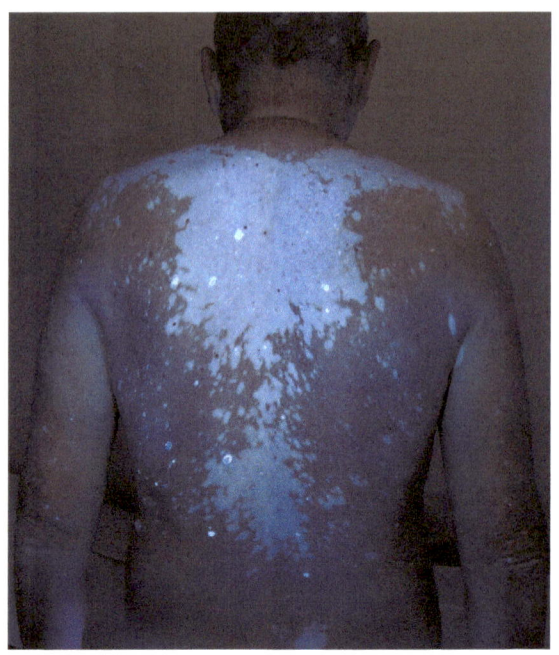

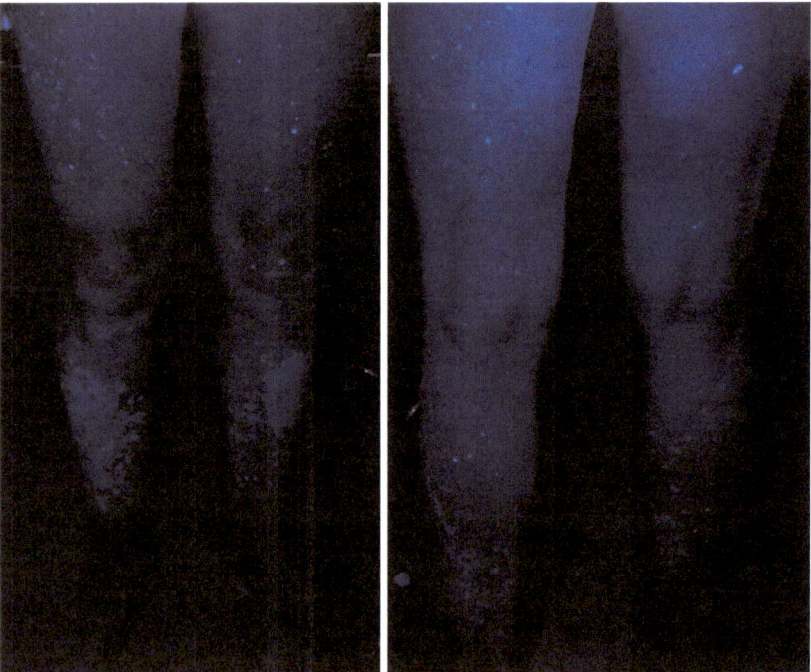

Fig. 37.2 On Wood's Lamp examination hypopigmented macules were well defined on the legs of
the man. Note the low fluorescence of the involved areas

Fig. 37.3 Lenticular macules on the abdomen of the patient. It can be seen the scar of the previous malignant melanoma

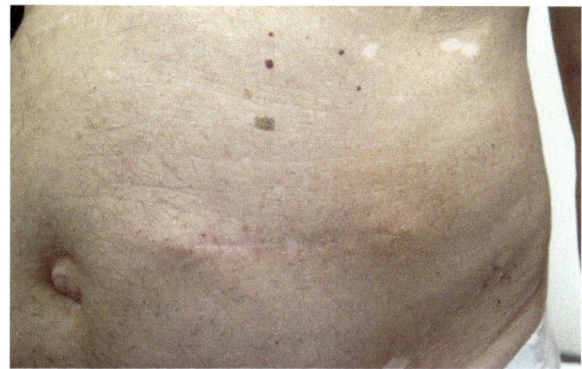

Diagnosis

Melanoma-associated leucoderma.

Discussion

Leucoderma is a condition characterised by depigmentation of the skin. When it appears in melanoma patients, it is called melanoma-associated leucoderma (MAL). First description of this phenomenon, which typically arises in distant sites from the area of the primary tumor—resulting in achromic patches resembling vitiligo-, dates back to the 1970s. MAL is considered an independent positive prognostic marker for melanoma patients in advanced stages [1].

Experimental investigations on this phenomenon showed that cytotoxic T lymphocytes recognize melanoma associated antigens shared also by non-neoplastic melanocytes [2]. Accordingly, presence of circulating autoantibodies directed toward melanocytes in melanoma and vitiligo patiens can be found. To date clear immunological or histological differences between the two pathologies have not been found in literature. Nevertheless clinical features of MAL can differentiate it from vitiligo. In fact melanoma-associated leucoderma is not usually associated with family history of vitiligo or other autoimmune disorders and the age of onset is higher (median age 55 years). In addition, MAL patients usually present flecked depigmented macules mainly located in photo-exposed areas instead of patches commonly found in vitiligo and koebnerization is usually absent.

Vitiligo-like depigmentation is also described during melanoma immunotherapy and target therapy and it is associated with a favorable prognosis [3]. Although this phenomenon is observed mainly in metastatic melanoma patients, it has been reported also in other metastatic tumors treated with immunotherapy [4].

The significance of this adverse events in metastatic cancer other than melanoma is still to be determined. Therapy of MAL is similar to the vitiligo one.

Vitiligo is an acquired chronic autoimmune disease characterized by well-defined achromatic macules of the skin, resulting in a loss of epidermal melanocytes [5]. This condition affects 2% of the world's population and it is frequently associated with psychological remarkable impact. Patients present a positive family history for vitiligo or other autoimmune diseases frequently. The onset of this condition is commonly in the youth, but the disease can arise at any age. Clinical classification distinguishes three major type of manifestation: focal vitiligo (FV), segmental vitiligo (SV) and non-segmental vitiligo (NSV). The etiopathology of vitiligo is complex and referred mainly to an autoimmune T cell reaction directed against melanocytes. Increased oxidative stress, imbalance of keratinocytes and dermal cells, impaired intercellular adhesion and genetic component contribute to the disease [6]. Koebner phenomenon is often present and many triggers cause the onset and progression of the disease such as sunburns, chemical substances and mechanical trauma. Vitiligo treatment is challenging and ranges over from local therapies— i.e. corticosteroids and calcineurin inhibitors-, narrow-band UVB therapy (NB-UVB), to surgical techniques in selected cases.

Pityriasis Alba is a benign skin disorder that commonly affects children and adolescents, expecially those with atopic dermatitis. This condition is characterized by hypochromic patches and macules, often sourmounted by fine scales. Sometimes it is accompained by itching sensation. It is a non specific dermatosis with a reduction of melanin without decreased melanocyte count in the basal layer. Manifestations resolve spontaneously, generally within 1 year. Ointments and topical corticosteroids can be useful to accelerate this process.

Post-inflammatory hypopigmentation can be triggered by some physical or mechanical trauma, laser-therapy and inflammatory conditions such as scleroderma, lupus eritematosus, expecially discoid variant. Diagnosis is facilitated by medical history and physical examination. The investigation of the underlying cause is necessary to set up the appropriate therapy.

Key Points

1. Leucoderma-associated melanoma is an autoimmune phenomenon that can occur in melanoma patients and it is considered a positive independent prognostic factor in advanced stages.
2. In front of the onset of hypopigmentary disorder in adults an accurate medical history and inspection of the skin is mandatory to exclude melanoma-associated leucoderma.
3. MAL is described as a relative common adverse event of immunotherapy in melanoma metastatic patients.

References

1. Quaglino P, Marenco F, Osella-Abate S, Cappello N, Ortoncelli M, Salomone B, et al. Vitiligo is an independent favourable prognostic factor in stage III and IV metastatic melanoma patients: results from a single-institution hospital-based observational cohort study. Ann Oncol. 2010 Feb;21(2):409–14.
2. Failla CM, Carbone ML, Fortes C, Pagnanelli G, D'Atri S. Melanoma and Vitiligo: in good company. Int J Mol Sci. 2019 Nov 15;20(22):5731.
3. Dousset L, Boniface K, Seneschal J. Vitiligo-like lesions occurring in patients receiving anti-programmed cell death-1 therapies. G Ital Dermatol Venereol. 2019 Aug;154(4):435–43.
4. Billon E, Walz J, Brunelle S, et al. Vitiligo adverse event observed in a patient with durable complete response after Nivolumab for metastatic renal cell carcinoma. Front Oncol. 2019 Oct 9;9:1033.
5. Boniface K, Seneschal J, Picardo M, Vitiligo TA. Focus on clinical aspects, Immunopathogenesis, and therapy. Clin Rev Allergy Immunol. 2018 Feb;54(1):52–67.
6. Delmas V, Larue L. Molecular and cellular basis of depigmentation in vitiligo patients. Exp Dermatol. 2019 Jun;28(6):662–6.

Chapter 38
A Pigmented Lesion with Pitfalls

Yasemin Yuyucu Karabulut, Eda Gökalp Satıcı, Mustafa Anıl Yılmaz, and Ümit Türsen

A 71-year-old man presented to the dermatology outpatient clinic because of pigmented lesions on his inguinal area. In the inguinal area, 5 cm diameter, verrucous pigmented lesion was observed dermoscopic examination of this lesion revealed fissures and ridges cerebriform appearance, hairpin blood vessels, and moth-eaten border (Fig. 38.1). Verrucous carcinoma and melanoma were considered and biopsy was taken.

Histopathological examination of the incisional biopsy revealed irregular acanthosis, mild hyperkeratosis as well as keratin plugs in the epidermis and skin biopsy was reported as seborrheic keratosis (Figs. 38.2 and 38.3).

When the patient developed a nodular structure in the middle of this verrucous lesion at the follow-up visit a month later, with increased suspicion of malignant melanoma re-biopsy was performed considering the presence of pigmentation and nodular structure. Histopathological examination of the biopsies revealed microscopic findings similar to the first biopsy and the new biopsy was interpreted as seborrheic keratosis, supporting the previous one (Fig. 38.4), and cryotherapy was applied to the lesion.

In the second month follow-up after cryotherapy, the lesion was seen to be substantially regressed (Fig. 38.5).

Y. Y. Karabulut · E. G. Satıcı
School of Medicine, Department of Pathology, Mersin University, Mersin, Turkey

M. A. Yılmaz · Ü. Türsen (✉)
School of Medicine, Department of Dermatology, Mersin University, Mersin, Turkey

T. Lotti et al. (eds.), *Clinical Cases in Melanoma*, Clinical Cases in Dermatology, https://doi.org/10.1007/978-3-030-50820-3_38

Fig. 38.1 The lesion is approximately 5 cm in diameter, hyperpigmented and contains nodular areas. Fissures and ridges cerebriform appearance, hairpin blood vessels, moth-eaten border were observed in dermoscopic examination

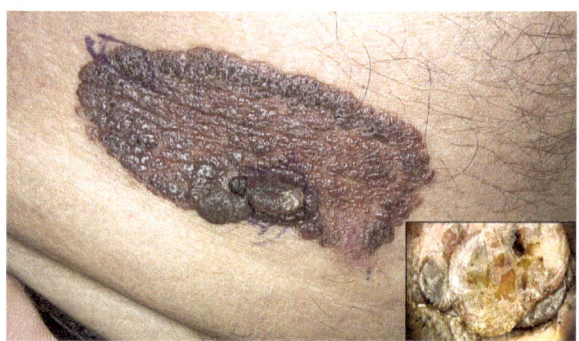

Fig. 38.2 Fig. 38.3: Histopathologically, hyperkeratosis, irregular acanthosis and keratin plugs were detected in the epidermis. (H&E, ×100)

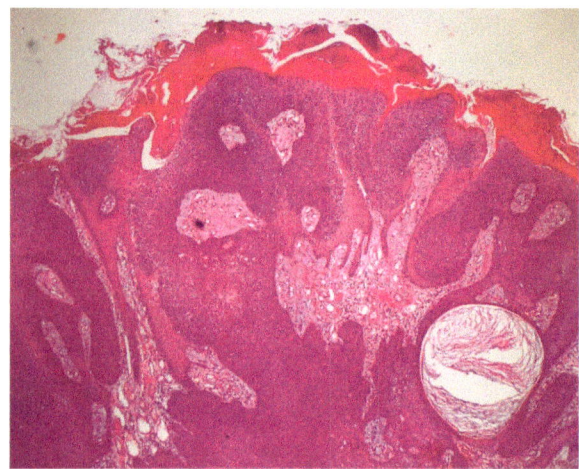

Fig. 38.3 Keratin plug in the epidermis (H&E, ×400)

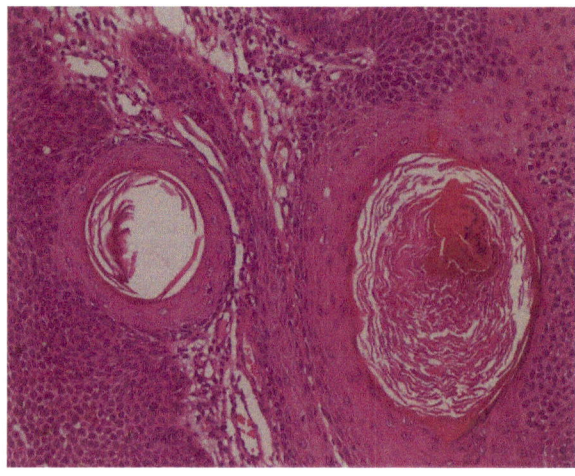

Fig. 38.4 Squamous
eddies and melanin
pigments in the epidermis.
(H&E, ×400)

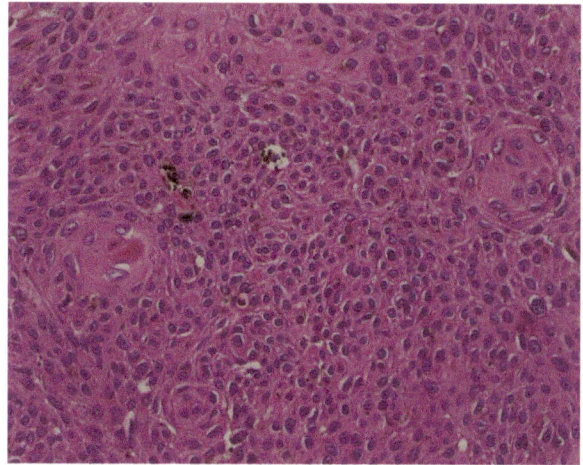

Fig. 38.5 Substantially
regressed lesion after
cryotherapy

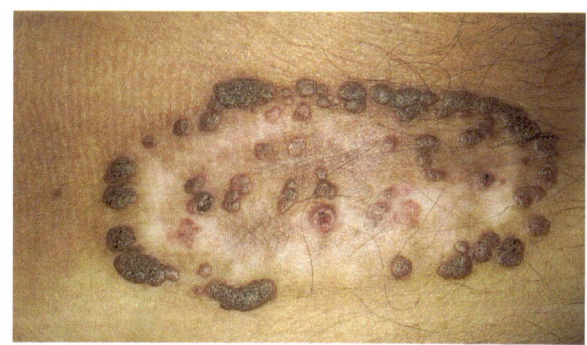

Based on the Case Description and the Photograph, What Is Your Diagnosis?

1. Malignant melanoma
2. Pigmented basal cell carcinoma
3. Verrucous melanoma
4. Seborrheic keratosis

Diagnosis

Seborrheic keratosis.

Discussion

Seborrheic keratosis is a benign skin neoplasm which is frequently seen in clinical practice. They are often located on the head, neck and chest, but they can be seen everywhere in the skin [1]. Clinical examination is sufficient in the diagnosis of most of them. Some pigmented seborrheic keratosis lesions can be confused clinically with malign skin tumors. Histopathological examination is mandatory in such cases.

Malignant melanoma, pigmented basal cell carcinoma, verrucous carcinoma and squamous cell carcinoma are among the most prominent malignant skin tumors mimicking pigmented seborrheic keratosis.

In a study by Tiffany Y. Chen et al., 4361 cases of seborrheic keratosis and seborrheic keratosis of irrites were discussed. Their histopathological examination revealed that 136 (3.1%) were malignant. Of these, 91 were reported as squamous cell carcinoma, 33 were basal cell carcinoma, and 12 were melanoma [2].

In another study, 402 lesions with 138 patients diagnosed as seborrheic keratosis were evaluated and 42 (10.44%) were reported to have dermoscopic criteria suggesting melanocytic origin [3].

One of the major dermoscopic pitfalls of seborrheic keratosis was reported to be malignant melanoma in a paper that drew attention to dermoscopy and pathology cooperation 308/5000 [4].

Melanoma and seborrheic keratosis are two different entities that can clinically mimic each other, but have very different prognosis and treatment options. Therefore, making this distinction is vital. Histopathological examination is the only option in the diagnosis of lesions suggesting both entities clinically.

Key Points

- Pigmented seborrheic keratoses may not be clinically indistinguishable from malignant melanoma.
- Histopathological evaluation is very valuable when dermatological examination and dermoscopy findings are insufficient to differentiate seborrheic keratosis and malignant melanoma.

References

1. Hafner C, Vogt T. Seborrheic keratosis. J Dtsch Dermatol Ges. 2008;6:664–77.
2. Chen TY, Morrison AO, Cockerell CJ. Cutaneous malignancies simulating seborrheic keratoses: an underappreciated phenomenon? J Cutan Pathol. 2017;44:747–8.

3. De Giorgi V, Massi D, Stante M, Carli P. False "melanocytic" parameters shown by pigmented seborrheic keratoses: a finding which is not uncommon in dermoscopy. Dermatol Surg. 2002;28(8):776–9.
4. Minagawa A. Dermoscopy–pathology relationship in seborrheic keratosis. J Dermatol. 2017;44(5):518–24.

Chapter 39
A Whitish Nodule on the Neck

Funda Bozkurt, Yasemin Yuyucu Karabulut, and Ümit Türsen

A 50-year-old male patient presented to a dermatology clinic with a mass on the neck (Fig. 39.1) and a biopsy was performed from the lesion.

The lesion, which was reported as a skin appendages tumor that cannot be distinguished from hydroadenoma/hydrocarcinoma in the outer center, was consulted to our laboratory.

In histopathological examination, nodular growth pattern was detected in the tumor (Fig. 39.2). It's consisted of atypical cells with large eosinophilic cytoplasm, big nucleus, prominent nucleoli. Cells with clear cytoplasm were also observed in some areas. Squamous differentiation, focal necrosis and increased mitosis were detected in the tumor (Fig. 39.3).

Immunohistochemical evaluation revealed focal pale cytoplasmic staining with polyclonal CEA in tumor cells, and no immunreactivity was observed with p63,

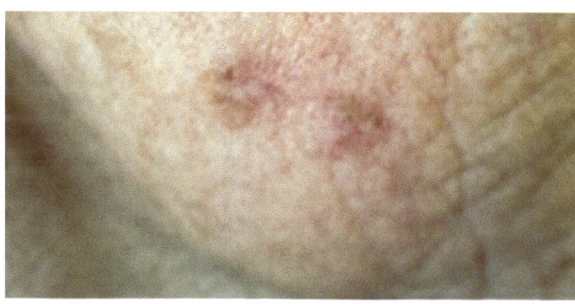

Fig. 39.1 Tumoral mass on the neck

F. Bozkurt · Y. Y. Karabulut
School of Medicine, Department of Pathology, Mersin University, Mersin, Turkey

Ü. Türsen (✉)
School of Medicine, Department of Dermatology, Mersin University, Mersin, Turkey

© The Editor(s) (if applicable) and The Author(s), under exclusive license to Springer Nature Switzerland AG 2020
T. Lotti et al. (eds.), *Clinical Cases in Melanoma*,
Clinical Cases in Dermatology, https://doi.org/10.1007/978-3-030-50820-3_39

Fig. 39.2 Tumoral lesion showing nodular growth pattern (H&E ×40)

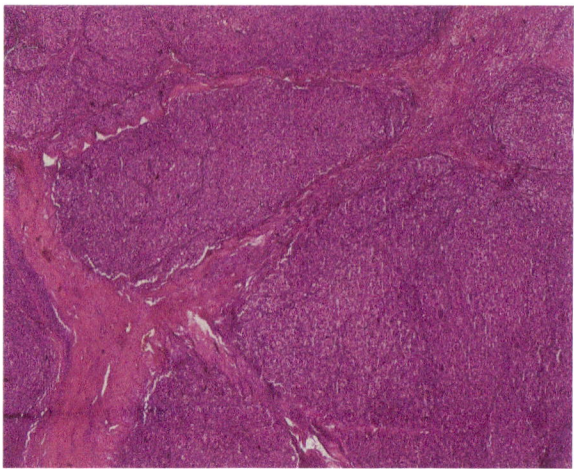

Fig. 39.3 Tumor cells with eosinophilic cytoplasm, large nuclei and increased mitosis (H&E ×400)

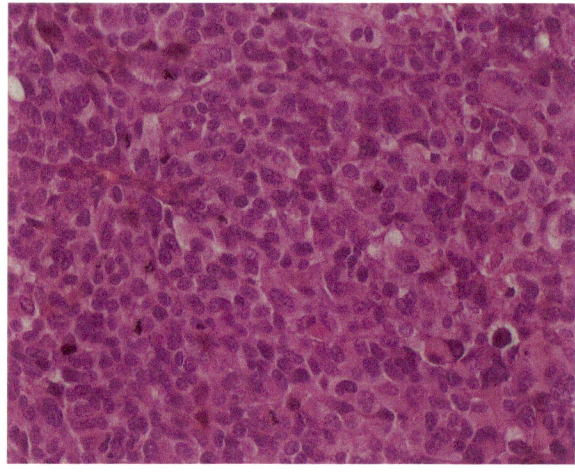

cytokeratin 20, bereb4, EMA, cytokeratin 7 and cytokeratin 19. The proliferative activity index with Ki-67 was 60%. With the findings of nuclear atypia, frequent mitosis and necrotic focus, it's reported as atypical hydroadenoma could not be excluded, excision is recommended for definitive diagnosis.

Within a few days total excision of the lesion was performed. On macroscopic examination, a nodular lesion with a size of 7 × 4 cm was observed. Atypical cells, forming solid layers, with nucleolar prominence was determined in microscopic examination (Fig. 39.4). The tumor cells were negative with HMB45, Panscytokeratin, Cytokeratin 7, EMA, Desmin, Cyclin D1, CD31, CD34, CD99, CD10, but cytoplasmic staining was detected with S100 (Fig. 39.5) and Melan-A (Fig. 39.6). And the case was reported as amelanotic malignant melanoma.

Fig. 39.4 Atypical cells, forming solid layers (H&E ×40)

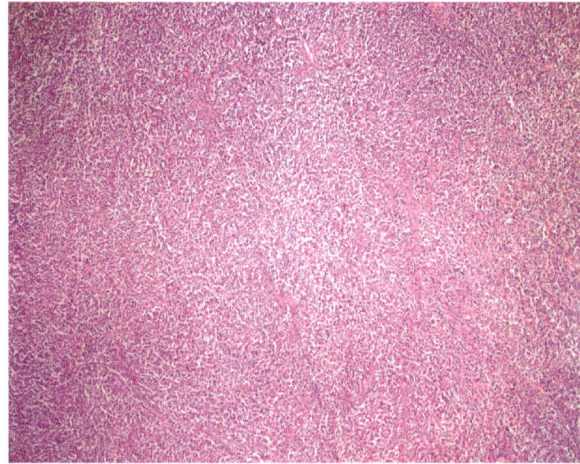

Fig. 39.5 Strong cytoplasmic staining with S100 (×40)

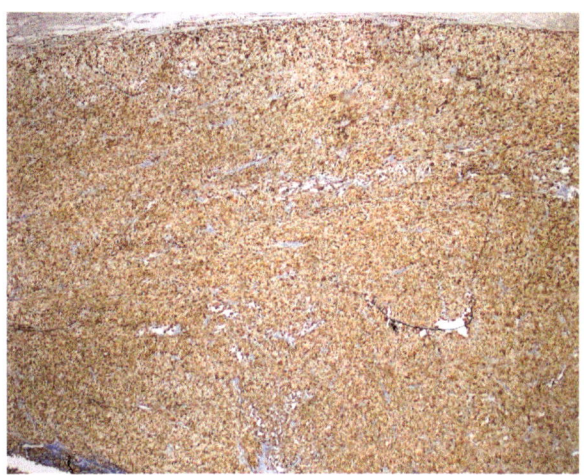

Clark invasion depth was determined as V, Breslow thickness was more than 4 mm. Pigmentation, ulceration, satellite nodule and perineural invasion were not observed in the tumor but vascular invasion was detected. Pet CT for systemic screening showed multiple metastatic nodular lesions in the bilateral lungs.

Based on the Case Description and the Photograph, What Is Your Diagnosis?

1. Basal cell carcinoma
2. Squamous cell carcinoma

Fig. 39.6 Strong
cytoplasmic staining with
Melan-A (×200)

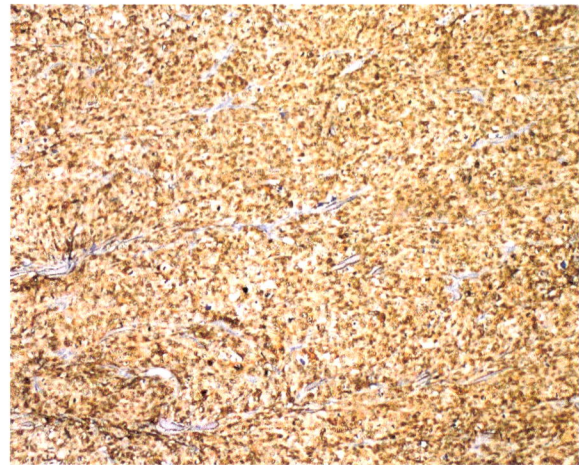

3. Nodular hidradenoma
4. Malignant nodular hidradenoma
5. Amelanotic melanoma

Diagnosis

Amelanotic melanoma.

Discussion

Amelanotic melanoma constitutes 2–8% of all melanomas and represents an atypical form that cannot be easily recognized as malignant melanoma [1, 2]. There are
two different models that explain the origin of amelanotic melanoma. First, amelanotic melanoma is claimed to be the poorly differentiated subtype of conventional
melanoma. Second, amelanotic melanoma is thought to be a dedifferentiated melanoma. However, in the literature, it has been shown that melanin deficiency in these
tumors is not caused by dedifferentiation or deficiency of melanin producing
enzymes. It has been determined that amelanotic melanoma tumor cells maintain
their melanocytic identity. These findings suggest that it is a third model that gained
the ability to form different phenotypes in the pathogenesis of amelanotic melanoma [3].

Histological evaluation with immunohistochemical staining is the gold standard
in the diagnosis of amelanotic melanoma [4]. Frequently used biomarkers are S100,
HMB-45, Melan-A, tyrosinase, MITF and Ki-67 [5].

Amelanotic melanoma in non-acral areas are most often confused with benign melanocytic lesions, such as basal cell carcinoma, squamous cell carcinoma, Bowen's disease, keratoacanthoma, seborrheic keratosis, pyogenic granuloma, dermatofibroma or dermatitis [3, 6, 7]. Other rare differential diagnoses reported include malignant nodular hidradenoma, nevus depigmentosus, granuloma annulare, Merkel cell carcinoma, and atypical fibrohistiocytic lesions [8, 9].

Amelanotic melanoma can mimic many benign or malignant conditions. They are usually diagnosed at an advanced stage due to delayed diagnosis and their prognosis is poor.

Key Points

- Amelanotic melanoma can mimic many benign and malignant entities clinically and histopathologically.
- Histological evaluation with immunohistochemical staining is the gold standard in the diagnosis of amelanotic melanoma.
- Clinicians and pathologists should keep in mind that amelanotic melanoma can occur with different clinical and morphological findings. In the differential diagnosis of suspicious lesions, amelanotic melanoma should consider.

References

1. Jaimes N, Braun RP, Thomas L, Marghoob AA. Clinical and dermoscopic characteristics of amelanotic melanomas that are not of the nodular subtype. J Eur Acad Dermatol Venereol. 2012;26:591–6.
2. McClain SE, Mayo KB, Shada AL, et al. Amelanotic melanomas presenting as red skin lesions: a diagnostic challenge with potentially lethal consequences. Int J Dermatol. 2012;51:420–6.
3. Cheung WL, Patel RR, Leonard A, Firoz B, Meehan SA. Amelanotic melanoma: a detailed morphologic analysis with clinicopathologic correlation of 75 cases. J Cutan Pathol. 2012;39(1):33–9.
4. Detrixhe A, Libon F, Mansuy M, Nikkels-Tassoudji N, Rorive A, Arrese JE, et al. Melanoma masquerading as nonmelanocytic lesions. Melanoma Res. 2016;26:631–4.
5. Ohsie SJ, Sarantopoulos GP, Cochran AJ, Binder SW. Immunohistochemical characteristics of melanoma. J Cutan Pathol. 2008;35:433–44.
6. Dainichi T, Kobayashi C, Fujita S, Shiramizu K, Ishiko T, Kiryu H, et al. Interdigital amelanotic spindle-cell melanoma mimicking an inflammatory process due to dermatophytosis. J Dermatol. 2007;34:716–9.
7. Soon SL, Solomon AR Jr, Papadopoulos D, Murray DR, McAlpine B, Washington CV. Acral lentiginous melanoma mimicking benign disease: the Emory experience. J Am Acad Dermatol. 2003;48:183–8.
8. Rahbari H, Nabai H, Mehregan AH, Mehregan DA, Mehregan DR, Lipinski J. Amelanotic lentigo maligna melanoma: a diagnostic conundrum –presentation of four new cases. Cancer. 1996;77:2052–7.
9. Satter EK. Amelanotic melanoma mimicking an atypical fibrohistiocytic lesion. Am J Dermatopathol. 2015;37:505–7.

Chapter 40
An Elderly Male with an Exophytic Ulcerated Lesion on Toenail

Tugba Kevser Uzuncakmak, Ozge Askin, Umit Tursen, and Zekayi Kutlubay

A 76-year-old male presented to the dermatology department with a 6 months history of rapidly growing lesion on his right toenail (Fig. 40.1). He administered to different dermatology clinics and was treated as a complicated ingrown toenail and onychomycosis.

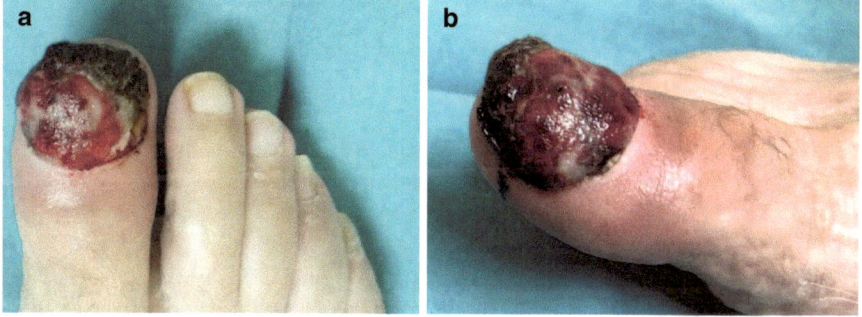

Fig. 40.1 (**a, b**) A rapidly growing exophytic and ulcerated tumoral lesion on right toenail

T. K. Uzuncakmak · O. Askin · Z. Kutlubay
Cerrahpasa Medical Faculty Department of Dermatology, Istanbul University-Cerrahpasa, Istanbul, Turkey

U. Tursen (✉)
Mersin University Medical Faculty Department of Dermatology, Mersin, Turkey

189

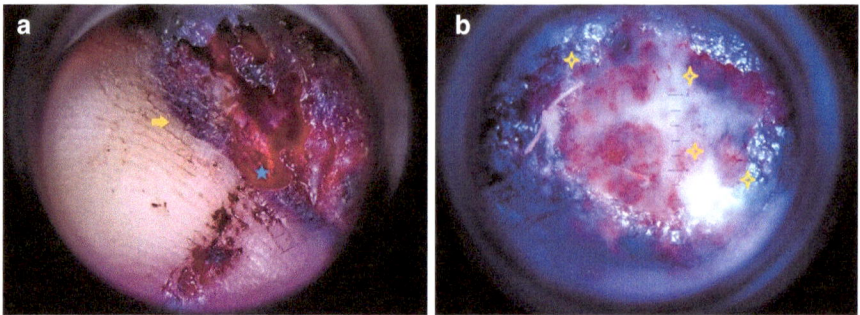

Fig. 40.2 (**a, b**) Dermoscopically, hemorrhagic crusts, active hemorrhage, polymorphic vessels on the lesion and parallel ridge pattern on distal fold of the nail. Yellow arrow: parallel ridge pattern. Blue star: hemorrhage. Yellow stars: lineer, glomeruler, branched polymorphic vessels

Based on the Case Description and the Photograph, What Is Your Diagnosis?

1. Squamous cell carcinoma
2. Onychomatricoma
3. Melanoma
4. Pyogenic granuloma
5. Kaposi sarcoma

On dermoscopic examination hemorrhagic crusts, active hemorrhage and polymorphic vessels were detected on the lesion, also parallel ridge pattern was positive on distal nail fold (Fig. 40.2).

An incisional biopsy was performed for initial diagnosis. Histopathologically, marked atypical melanocytic proliferation was noted. Breslow thickness was 3.2 mm, mitoses was 10 mm² and no lymphovascular and perineural invasion were detected. He was referred to Plastic Surgery Department for total excision and sentinel lymph node biopsy (Fig. 40.3).

Diagnosis

Subungual melanoma.

Discussion

Subungual melanoma (SUM) is a rare type of melanoma accounting for approximately 0.7–3% of all melanomas [1]. It was first described by *Hutchinson* in 1886 and has a worse prognosis compared to other melanoma types, probably due to the

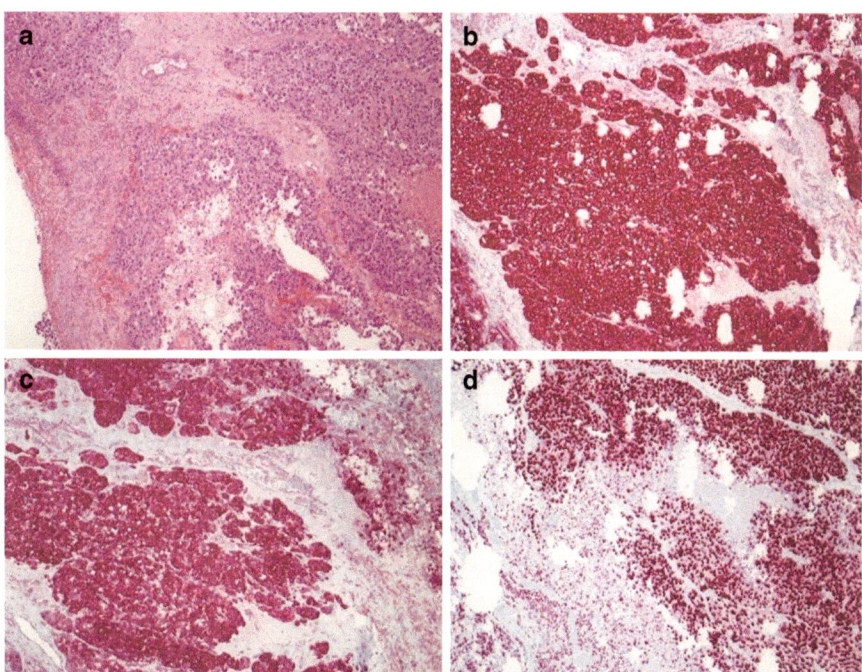

Fig. 40.3 (**a**) Marked atypia with pleomorphic nuclei with large eosinophilic nucleoli, necrosis and hemorrage surrounding tumoral infiltration (H&E, ×100), (**b**) Positive staining with HMB45 (×100), (**c**) Positive staining with MART1 (×100), (**d**) Positive staining with SOX10 (×100)

diagnosis at a more advanced stage. In that, the time between onset of symptoms and diagnosis was reported to range from 1.4 to 2.2 years in epidemiological studies [2]. The disease onset is more common between the fifth and seventh decades of life and represents no predilection for sex. SUM lesions begin in the skin at the border or just below the nail and present as nail pigmentation. Clinically it presents as longitudinal melanonychia but may also mimick various other dermatoses such as subungual haematoma, paronychia, pyogenic granuloma and onychomycosis that may lead to diagnostic delays and compromise prognosis [3]. In clinical studies just 20% of SUMs were diagnosed at stage 1 and were reported to be more common in hands. While the majority of hand SUM had a Breslow ≤1 mm while most of foot SUM had a Breslow >1 mm at the time of diagnosis [1, 2]. The survival rate in patients with an ulcerated tumor was also reported to be lower than in those with a tumor without ulceration at the same stage.

The pathogenesis of SUM has not yet been clarified. It is not associated with sun exposure, and BRAF mutations are not common in this type of melanoma. The genetic mutations including PIK3CA, STK11, EGFR, FGFR3, CDK4, cyclin D1 and PTPN11 genes have shown in a higher frequency of copy number aberrations in SUM lesions [4]. Trauma was also reported to have a potential role on induction of reactive hyperplasia of the nail unit melanocytes was but this hypothesis was supported only in a few studies [1].

The treatment of SUM depends on tumor thickness, lymphovascular and peri-neural invasion status. Classical treatment is digit amputation; but there is a challenge about preserving esthetis and functionality of the affected digit while providing tumor free margins. More over nonamputative conservative surgeries may be performed in insitu lesions and lesions having thin and intermediate depth [2]. Better aesthetic and functional results have been in small case series without affecting overall survival or recurrence free survival.

Key Points

• Subungual melanoma is a rare type of melanoma which is more common between the fifth and seventh decades of life.
• Subungual melanoma lesions begin in the skin at the border or just below the nail and present as nail pigmentation that may mimick various other dermatoses such as subungual haematoma, paronychia, pyogenic granuloma and onychomycosis, clinically.

References

1. Kostaki M, Plaka M, Stergiopoulou A, et al. Subungual melanoma: the experience of a Greek melanoma reference center from 2003 to 2018. J Eur Acad Dermatol Venereol. 2020 Jan 16;34:e231–4. https://doi.org/10.1111/jdv.16193.
2. Nunes LF, Mendes GLQ, Koifman RJ. Subungual melanoma: a retrospective cohort of 157 cases from Brazilian National Cancer Institute. J Surg Oncol. 2018;118:1142–9. https://doi.org/10.1002/jso.25242.
3. Finlay B, Ramachandren T, Hussey K, et al. Nodular melanoma presenting as an exophytic subungual mass. Scott Med J. 2018;63:32–4. https://doi.org/10.1177/0036933018755938.
4. Wollina U, Tempel S, Hansel G. Subungual melanoma: A single center series from Dresden. Dermatol Ther. 2019;32:e13032. https://doi.org/10.1111/dth.13032.

Chapter 41
A Man with a Painless Isolated Fingernail Dystrophy

Uwe Wollina

The 81-year-old male patient presented with a partial destruction of the nail plate of his fourth right digit. The lesion developed over 4 months. He reported no pain and bleeding. Hutchinson's sign was negative. The distal nail bed presented a hyperkeratotic firm nodule. There was no axillary lymphadenopathy.

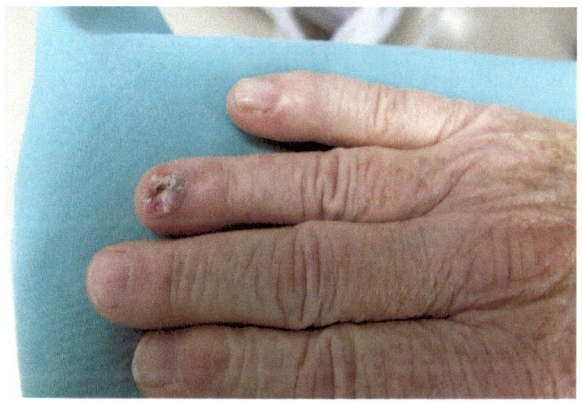

Initial presentation of a partial nail plate destruction on the fourth digit

U. Wollina (✉)
Department of Dermatology and Allergology, Municipal Hospital of Dresden,
Academic Teaching Hospital, Dresden, Germany
e-mail: Uwe.Wollina@klinikum-dresden.de

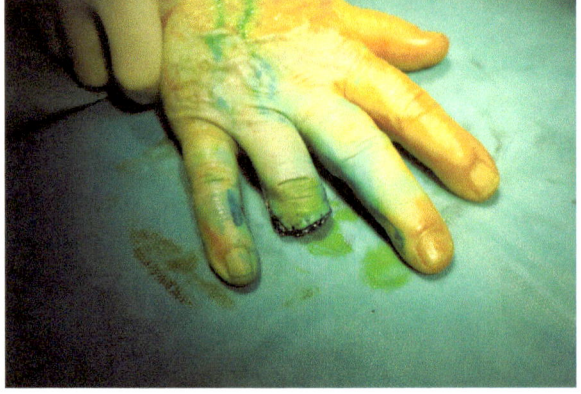

Operation situs after functional amputation

Based on the Case Description and the Photograph, What Is Your Diagnosis?

- Lichen planus of the nail bed
- Onychomycosis
- Acrolentiginous melanoma
- Bowen's disease of the nail bed
- Subungual warts.

Diagnosis

Acrolentiginous melanoma of the nail bed, Breslow index 2.48 mm, Clark level IV, pT3a pN0 (0/3sn) M0; perineural infiltration, lymphangiosis blastomatosa.

Discussion

The nail was investigated by naked eye and dermoscopy. Black or brown pigmentation was absent. A nail bed biopsy was taken to exclude an epithelial cancer. Histology revealed a mostly amelanotic acrolentiginous melanoma with both perineural infiltration and infiltration of lymphatic vessels. In cooperation with the hand surgeon a functional amputation of the distal digit was performed. In response to the reported tumor thickness of 2.48 mm a sentinel lymph node excision was performed. Three axillary lymph nodes were marked by Te, removed and histologically analyzed. All three were tumor negative. Healing after surgery was unremarkable. Staging by diagnostic ultrasound, magnetic resonance imaging of the head and computerized tomography of the trunk gave no hint of any metastatic spread.

Any uncertain nail disorder warrants a nail biopsy to exclude a malignancy. A negative Hutchinson's sign and a missing pigmentation of the nail bed or nail folds do not exclude melanoma diagnosis [1].

Acrolentiginous melanoma is one of the four major subtypes of cutaneous melanoma. In a multivariate analysis of 2050 patients, age ($P = 0.006$), ulceration ($P = 0.013$), tumor thickness ($P < 0.001$), and tumor spread ($P < 0.001$) have been identified as significant prognostic factors for disease free survival, whereas sex, nevus and level of invasion were not independent factors [2].

Due to a delay in diagnosis acrolentiginous melanoma is thought to have an unfavorable prognosis [3].

Key Points

- Any uncertain nail disorder should be investigated histologically.
- Subungual melanoma is one of the four major subtypes of cutaneous melanoma.
- Subungual melanoma has the same prognostic markers as the other types of cutaneous melanoma.
- Delay of diagnosis is the major factor leading to a more unfavorable prognosis.

References

1. Wollina U, Tempel S, Hansel G. Subungual melanoma: a single center series from Dresden. Dermatol Ther. 2019;32(5):e13032.
2. Teramoto Y, Keim U, Gesierich A, Schuler G, Fiedler E, Tüting T, et al. Acral lentiginous melanoma: a skin cancer with unfavourable prognostic features. A study of the German central malignant melanoma registry (CMMR) in 2050 patients. Br J Dermatol. 2018;178(2):443–51.
3. Goydos JS, Shoen SL. Acral Lentiginous Melanoma. Cancer Treat Res. 2016;167:321–9.

Chapter 42
A Man with an Oozing Nodule and a Black Plaque

Uwe Wollina and Gesina Hansel

The 46-year-old male patient presented with an oozing and malodourous nodule as large as a hen's egg on the abdominal skin. He presented because of staining of the underwear and the odor. He did not complain about other symptoms. His medical history was otherwise unremarkable.

On examination we observed a large exophytic flesh-colored nodule and medially from it two plaques—one also flesh-colored, the other one black—on the right side of his abdomen. Furthermore, we noted two subcutaneous nodules nearby.

The laboratory analysis revealed a slight neutrophilia of 76.8% (normal range 35–75%), lymphopenia of 15.0% (20–45%), ASAT 1.24 µkat/L (<0.85 µkat/L), LDH 6.55 µkat/L (2.25–3.75 µkat/L).

U. Wollina (✉) · G. Hansel
Department of Dermatology and Allergology, Municipal Hospital of Dresden, Academic Teaching Hospital, Dresden, Germany
e-mail: Uwe.Wollina@klinikum-dresden.de

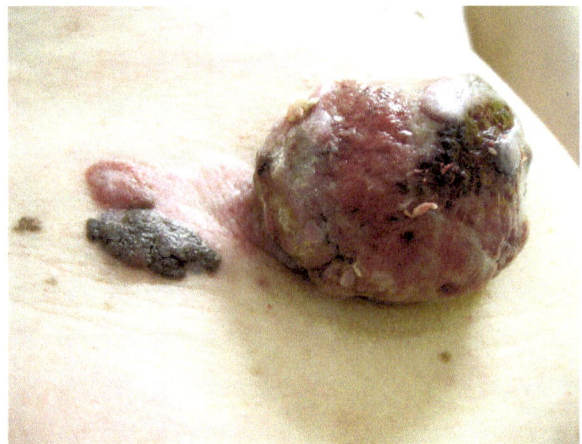

Initial presentation of a large exophytic flesh-colored nodules and two plaques

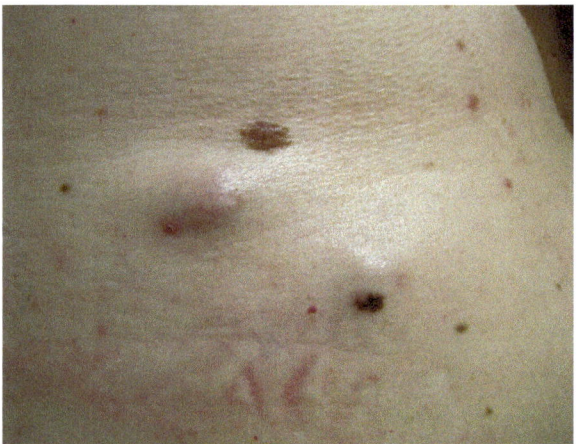

Two subcutaneous firm nodules

Based on the Case Description and the Photograph, What Is Your Diagnosis?

- Liposarcoma.
- B-cell lymphoma, leg type.
- Amelanotic melanoma.
- Melanoma and sarcoma

Diagnosis
Ulcerated nodular melanoma, Breslow index 35 mm, Clark level V (large tumor) plus superficial spreading melanoma, Breslow index undefined, Clark level II plus. Metastases were detected: two in-transit metastases, four axillary lymph node metastases. This results in tumor stage pT4b, pN3 (4/4), cM0—stage IIIC.

Discussion

Today most patients with melanoma present in early stages [1]. In Germany, the majority of new patients present in tumor stage I what results in a better prognosis [2]. Nevertheless, the number of melanomas thicker than 2 mm remains relatively stable.

This patient presented with two primary melanomas—a nodular amelanotic and a superficial spreading one close by. His S100 level on first presentation was 0.384 µg/ L. In histopathology the amelanotic tumor expressed Mart-1 and S-100. The tumor was BRAF positive.

Tumor staging detected two in-transit and four axillary lymph node metastases on primary examination. MRI scan of the cerebrum was unremarkable. CT scan of the trunk revealed pulmonary lesions suspicious of metastases. We started with nivolumab twice a month from June 2016 to April 2018. During this time four subcutaneous metastases were surgically removed. In January 2017, a new axillary metastasis was detected, and lymph node dissection had been performed with two positive nodes out of eight. In April 2017 an osseous metastasis of the 12th rib could be detected in a PET-CT scan. We initiated zoledronic acid infusions once a month.

In May 2018, we switched the treatment to pembrolizumab with regression of the osseous metastasis. Due to progressive edema of arms and legs, pembolizumab was abrogated in January 2019 and nivolumab was re-initiated. The treatment resulted in a complete remission and was stopped in March. Re-staging in August confirmed the complete remission. Immune mediated arthritis developed and was treated by low dose oral prednisolone.

The course of this patients underlines the greater opportunities in tumor control with targeted and immune therapies that become available recently in combination with surgical removal of metastases [1, 3, 4]. Despite a worse prognosis at the first visit (tumor thickness high, tumor amelanotic and ulcerated, LDH increased) the patient survived until now 40 months with tumor therapy and achieved a complete remission. He will continue a follow-up in the skin cancer center.

Key Points
- Amelanotic melanoma is a challenge for clinical diagnosis.
- Tumor prognosis depends upon tumor thickness, ulceration and tumor stage at first presentation.
- Tumor prognosis has become improved with immune and targeted therapies.
- The new treatment options need a close monitoring for possible adverse events.

References

1. Schadendorf D, van Akkooi ACJ, Berking C, Griewank KG, Gutzmer R, Hauschild A, Stang A, Roesch A, Ugurel S. Melanoma. Lancet. 2018;392(10151):971–84.
2. Hübner J, Eisemann N, Brunßen A, Katalinic A. Skin cancer screening in Germany: review after ten years. Bundesgesundheitsblatt Gesundheitsforschung Gesundheitsschutz. 2018;61(12):1536–43.
3. Bomar L, Senithilnathan A, Ahn C. Systemic therapies for advanced melanoma. Dermatol Clin. 2019;37(4):409–23.
4. Wollina U, Brzezinski P. The value of metastasectomy in stage IV cutaneous melanoma. Wien Med Wochenschr. 2019;169(13–14):331–8.

Chapter 43
A Painful Dyschromic Prepatellar Tumor

Uwe Wollina

A 59-year-old male patient was hospitalized due to an acute erysipelas (cellulitis) of his right lower leg. He was treated by intravenous penicillin G 10 mega units every 8 h. During his stay in the hospital he developed a painful prepatellar tumor (nodule) on the same leg. His medical history was positive for diabetes, hypertension, hepatic hemangiomas, sigma diverticulosis, and mixed alcoholic and metabolic liver cirrhosis. He was treated with amlodipine, atorvastatin, hydrochlorothiazide, olmesartan, pantoprazole, and propranolol.

Based on the Case Description and the Photograph, What Is Your Diagnosis?

1. Gout tophus.
2. Bursitis.
3. Abscess.
4. Hematoma.
5. Angiosarcoma.

U. Wollina (✉)
Department of Dermatology and Allergology, Municipal Hospital of Dresden, Academic Teaching Hospital, Dresden, Germany
e-mail: Uwe.Wollina@klinikum-dresden.de

201
T. Lotti et al. (eds.), *Clinical Cases in Melanoma*,
Clinical Cases in Dermatology, https://doi.org/10.1007/978-3-030-50820-3_43

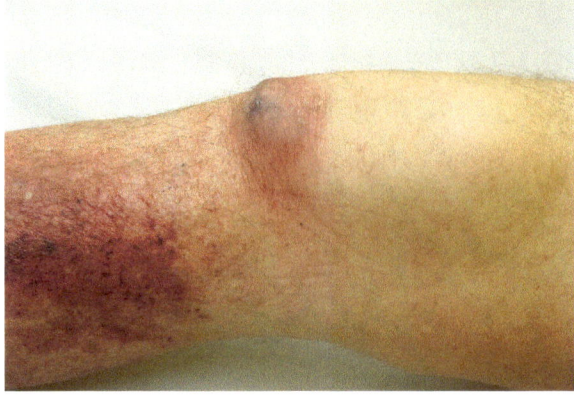

Painful prepatellar nodule, remnants of erysipelas are visible on the lower leg

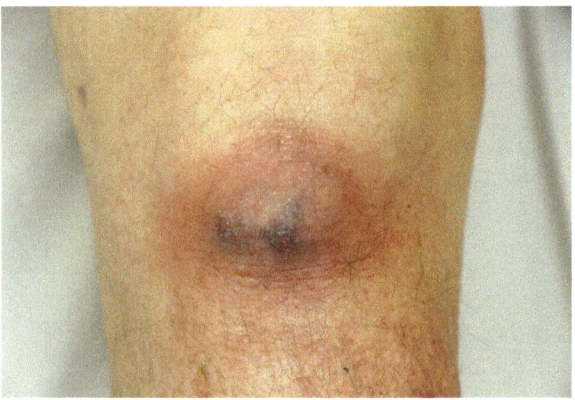

Prepatellar painful nodule with red and bluish coloration

Diagnosis
Gout Tophus.

Discussion

The patients presented a painful swelling on the right knee with redness and some bluish hyperpigmentation. During the course, we observed a spontaneous "putride", crumbly secretion. An orthopedic council and an X-ray of the knee excluded the bursitis. Duplex sonography of the leg veins remained normal.

Laboratory investigations revealed a C-reactive protein of 64.2 mg/L (normal range < 5 mg/L). Leukocytes were 19.75 Gpt/L (3.8–11.0 Gpt/L), hemoglobin was 8.0 mmol/L (8.6–12.1 mmol/L). Uric acid was 159 μmol/L (200–420 μmol/L). Gamma-globulins were 53.6% (8.0–15.8%).

Microbiologic swabs were negative.

We initiated pain management with oxycodon hydrochloride opened the tophus surgically, removed the whitish crumbly material and continued antibiosis. The bluish color was due to hemorrhages. To prevent thrombosis we gave certoparin sodium 3 × 8000 IU per day.

The diagnosis was a hemorrhagic gouty tophus. It healed within 5 days.

Gout is the most common type of arthritis caused by the deposition of monosodium urate crystals in or close to the joints. The world-wide prevalence is higher in industrialized countries with up to 10%, while the reported incidence ranges from 0.3 to 6 cases per 1000 person-years [1].

The tophus is a clinical symptom of advanced gout. Histologically, gouty tophi resemble foreign body granulomas. Extracellular trap formation by neutrophils interacting with monosodium urate crystals are essential for tophus formation. Tophaceous gout becomes more frequent with a longer history of untreated hyperuricemia. In case of renal disease, however, tophi can occur also at an early stage [2].

Treatment includes nonsteroidal anti-inflammatory drugs (NSAID), colchicine or prednisolone in acute flares and urate-lowering drugs like allopurinol, benzbromanone, febuxostat or pegloticase. In some cases, surgery is helpful [2–4]. In the present patient hepatic disease limited the use of NSAID. Therefore, we decided to use oxycodone and surgery. Microsopy confirmed urate monosodium crystals.

Gout is a part of the metabolic syndrome seen in the present patient. The low level of uric acid does not argue against a gouty tophus [5].

Key Points
- Gout is a common disorder in industrialized countries.
- Gouty tophus is a symptom of advanced disease.
- Treatment is often conservative, but sometimes surgery is helpful.

References

1. Kuo CF, Grainge MJ, Zhang W, Doherty M. Global epidemiology of gout: prevalence, incidence and risk factors. Nat Rev Rheumatol. 2015;11(11):649–62.
2. Chhana A, Dalbeth N. The gouty tophus: a review. Curr Rheumatol Rep. 2015;17(3):19.
3. Chokoeva AA, Tchernev G, Patterson JW, Lotti T, Wollina U. Acute overnight painful swelling of a finger. J Biol Regul Homeost Agents. 2015;29(1 Suppl):1–3.
4. Bouras T, Gandhi M, Barnett A. Diagnosis and treatment of patellar tendon gouty tophus: a case report. Surg J (N Y). 2019;5(2):e46–9.
5. Seth R, Kydd AS, Buchbinder R, Bombardier C, Edwards CJ. Allopurinol for chronic gout. Cochrane Database Syst Rev. 2014;10:CD006077.

Chapter 44
A Recalcitrant Onychomycosis

Uwe Wollina, Gesina Hansel, and Sven Tempel

A 45-year-old female patient presented in 2012 in a private clinic with a dystrophic thumb nail suggestive of an onychomycosis. She reported no trauma or pain. Mycologic investigations of nail clippings were performed for diagnostics and a combined topical and oral antimycotic therapy with terbinafine was initiated. When the patients returned after 3 months, no changes were noted, therefore a first nail biopsy was performed and sent to a pathology laboratory. The lab report gave no hints for any malignancy. Because of suspicion of an underlying pathology, the patient was referred to the hospital for a second opinion.

The patient was otherwise healthy. She took no medical drugs. She had no professional exposure to wet work or contact to animals.

On examination we observed a complete yellowish nail dystrophy of the left thumb. The cuticle was destroyed, but there was no nail fold edema, no Hutchinson sign. All the other nails remained unaffected. Clinically no lymphadenopathy was evident. The patient was in a good general condition. We performed a second nail bed biopsy.

U. Wollina (✉) · G. Hansel
Department of Dermatology and Allergology, Municipal Hospital of Dresden, Academic Teaching Hospital, Dresden, Germany
e-mail: Uwe.Wollina@klinikum-dresden.de; Gesina.Hansel@klinikum-dresden.de

S. Tempel
Department of Trauma, Reconstructive and Hand Surgery, Municipal Hospital of Dresden, Academic Teaching Hospital, Dresden, Germany
e-mail: Sven.Tempel@klinikum-dresden.de

T. Lotti et al. (eds.), *Clinical Cases in Melanoma*,
Clinical Cases in Dermatology, https://doi.org/10.1007/978-3-030-50820-3_44

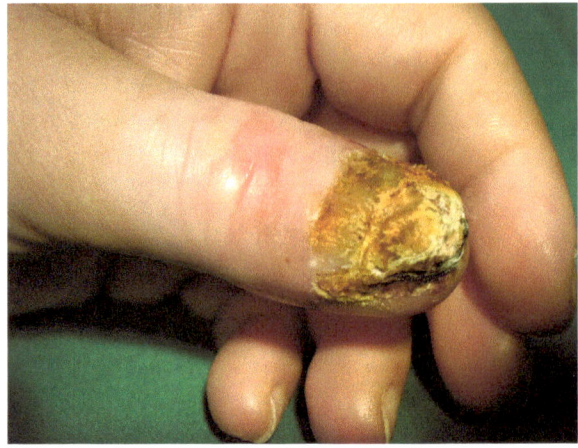

Initial presentation of a dystrophic, distally thickened yellowish thumb nail

Based on the Case Description and the Photograph, What Is Your Diagnosis?

- Candidiasis of the nail.
- Bowen's disease of the nail bed.
- Traumatic onychodystrophy.
- Acrolentiginous melanoma.

Diagnosis
Acrolentiginous melanoma, Breslow index 5.0 mm, Clark level IV; tumor stage pT4b, cN0, cM0—stage IIC.

Discussion

In case of disorders recalcitrant to the usual treatment the diagnosis has to be re-considered. The first working diagnosis was onychomycosis and terbinafine was prescribed. Terbinafine is less effective in cure of yeast infections compared to azoles [1], but the patient was not a person at risk for candida-infections. She had no diabetes or chronic mucocutaneous candidiasis—an immunodeficient disorder of the interleukin-17 pathway [2]. Recently, terbinafine-resistant variants of Trichophyton mentagrophytes have been identified in India. The species exert a mutation of the internal transcribed spacer (ITS). This Indian ITS phenotype is associated with terbinafine resistance [3, 4]. However, the patient had never visited the Indian subcontinent.

Bowen's disease or squamous cell carcinoma of the nail may present with a similar phenotype [5]. As a consequence, a nail (bed) biopsy is necessary. In the present patients the second biopsy revealed tumor cells of the spindle and epitheloid cell type infiltrating the mid-corium. The tumor was associated with a peripheral in situ-component. We performed a subtotal resection of the thumb with delayed Mohs surgery in cooperation with the hand surgeon in combination with sentinel lymph node excision of the left axilla. Histology ensured that the bone remained unaffected. However, the in situ-components reached the proximal resection margin. We performed a second excision that leads to tumor-free resection margins. Healing was unremarkable. The sentinel lymph node was tumor free. The melanoma was BRAF-wild-type. Laboratory investigations were unremarkable.

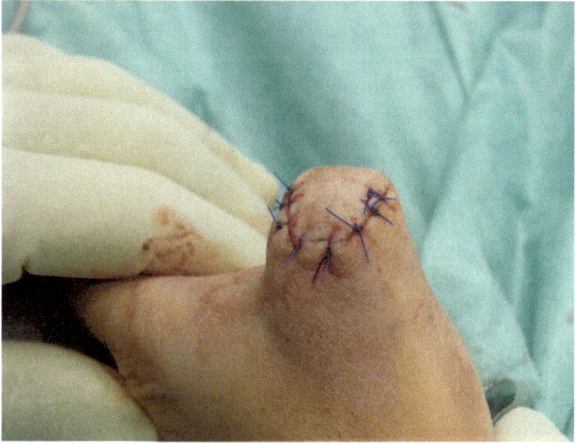

Operation situs after R0-resection

We initiated a low-dose subcutaneous therapy with interferon-alpha for 2 years. In November 2017 she developed an axillary lymph node metastasis, and subsequently and axilla dissection was performed with 5 of 8 positive nodes. We reintroduced the interferon therapy in January 2018. Until May 2018 she remained in complete remission. During a re-staging with MRI and PET-CT she presented with multiple metastases of abdominal lymph nodes, liver and bone. Interferon was stopped and a combined nivolumab and ipilimumab treatment was started in June. A grade III immune-mediated colitis led to hospitalization and treatment with infliximab and prednisolone. In November, re-staging recorder a progress of liver metastases but not further tumor spread. Therefore, selective internal yttrium-90 radioembolization therapy (SIRT) was recommended by the multidisciplinary tumor board and performed in January 2019 [6]. After recovery, bone metastases and a new axillary metastasis were treated by radiotherapy. In November, we reintroduced combined nivolumab/ ipilimumab therapy. In the CHECKMATE 67 trial, the overall survival at 5 years was 52% in the nivolumab-plus-ipilimumab group vs. 43% with ipilimumab alone [7].

Key Points

- Disorders not responding to a treatment according to guidelines have to be reconsidered.
- Recalcitrant nail disease warrants a nail bed biopsy.
- A negative Hutchinson's sign does not exclude nail bed melanoma.

References

1. Gamarra S, Morano S, Dudiuk C, Mancilla E, Nardin ME, de Los Angeles Méndez E, Garcia-Effron G. Epidemiology and antifungal susceptibilities of yeasts causing vulvovaginitis in a teaching hospital. Mycopathologia. 2014;178(3-4):251–8.
2. Okada S. CMCD: chronic Mucocutaneous candidiasis disease. Nihon Rinsho Meneki Gakkai Kaishi. 2017;40(2):109–17.
3. Nenoff P, Verma SB, Vasani R, Burmester A, Hipler UC, Wittig F, Krüger C, Nenoff K, Wiegand C, Saraswat A, Madhu R, Panda S, Das A, Kura M, Jain A, Koch D, Gräser Y, Uhrlaß S. The current Indian epidemic of superficial dermatophytosis due to Trichophyton mentagrophytes – a molecular study. Mycoses. 2019;62(4):336–56.
4. Süß A, Uhrlaß S, Ludes A, Verma SB, Monod M, Krüger C, Nenoff P. Extensive tinea corporis due to a terbinafine-resistant Trichophyton mentagrophytes isolate of the Indian genotype in a young infant from Bahrain in Germany. Hautarzt. 2019;70(11):888–96.
5. Wollina U. Bowen's disease of the nail apparatus: a series of 8 patients and a literature review. Wien Med Wochenschr. 2015;165(19-20):401–5.
6. Xing M, Prajapati HJ, Dhanasekaran R, Lawson DH, Kokabi N, Eaton BR, Kim HS. Selective internal Yttrium-90 Radioembolization therapy (90Y-SIRT) versus best supportive Care in Patients with Unresectable Metastatic Melanoma to the liver refractory to systemic therapy: safety and efficacy cohort study. Am J Clin Oncol. 2017;40(1):27–34.
7. Larkin J, Chiarion-Sileni V, Gonzalez R, Grob JJ, Rutkowski P, Lao CD, Cowey CL, Schadendorf D, Wagstaff J, Dummer R, Ferrucci PF, Smylie M, Hogg D, Hill A, Márquez-Rodas I, Haanen J, Guidoboni M, Maio M, Schöffski P, Carlino MS, Lebbé C, McArthur G, Ascierto PA, Daniels GA, Long GV, Bastholt L, Rizzo JI, Balogh A, Moshyk A, Hodi FS, Wolchok JD. Five-year survival with combined Nivolumab and Ipilimumab in advanced melanoma. N Engl J Med. 2019;381(16):1535–46.

Chapter 45
An Ulcerated Nodule on the Flank of an 80-year-old Woman

Uwe Wollina

The 80-year-old female patient presented with an ulcerated nodular tumor on her left flank in 2010. She reported no pain or burning sensations. The lesion was growing slowly for several months but started bleeding recently.

Her medical history was remarkable for cardiac insufficiency, bypass surgery 9 years ago and pacemaker implantation 5 years ago. She suffered from high blood pressure and diabetes mellitus type 2 treated orally.

On examination we observed a partially ulcerated exophytic flesh-colored nodule surrounded by a multicolored but ill-defined flat margin. Clinically no lymphadenopathy was evident. The patient was in a good general condition so far.

U. Wollina (✉)
Department of Dermatology and Allergology, Municipal Hospital of Dresden, Academic Teaching Hospital, Dresden, Germany
e-mail: Uwe.Wollina@klinikum-dresden.de

© The Editor(s) (if applicable) and The Author(s), under exclusive license to
Springer Nature Switzerland AG 2020
T. Lotti et al. (eds.), *Clinical Cases in Melanoma*,
Clinical Cases in Dermatology, https://doi.org/10.1007/978-3-030-50820-3_45

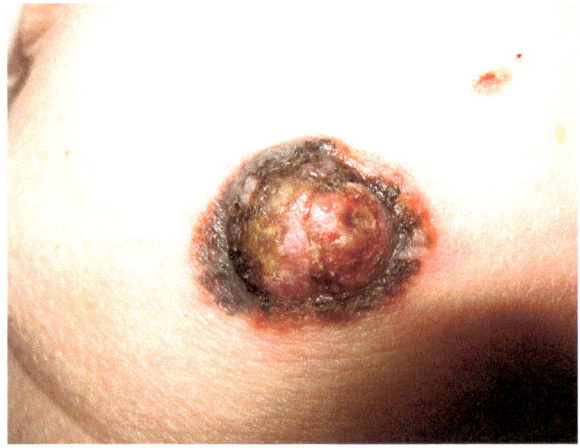

Initial presentation of a large exophytic flesh-colored nodules with a multicolored flat margin.

Based on the Case Description and the Photograph, What Is Your Diagnosis?

- Nodular melanoma.
- Bednar tumor.
- B-cell lymphoma.
- Superficial spreading melanoma with secondary nodular growth.
- Melanoma on a large melanocytic nevus.

Diagnosis

Superficial spreading melanoma with secondary nodular growth, partially ulcerated, Breslow index 4.25 mm, Clark level IV; tumor stage pT4b, cN0, cM0—stage IIC.

Discussion

Most melanomas develop de novo although melanoma and preexisting melanocytic nevus may be found closely together. Even in giant congenital melanocytic nevi, which have a higher risk for secondary development of melanoma, each melanoma cell develops sporadically and amplification of MYC might be a key event for melanoma development.

Secondary development of nodular melanoma on a primary superficial spreading melanoma illustrates a qualitative change in tumor behavior. Nodular melanoma is often associated with ulceration, rapid growth rate and high mitotic rate. They contribute substantially to melanoma-related mortality [1].

While superficial spreading melanoma shows a correlation to lighter skin types, nodular melanoma does not [2].

Our patient demonstrated an increased LDH of 4.62 μkat/ L (normal range 2.25–3.55 μkat/ L), S100 was 0.061 μg/ L. Imaging with diagnostic ultrasound (axilla and groin, abdomen) and thoracic X-ray did not find any signs suggestive for melanoma spread. Due to the advanced age and tumor thickness we renounced sentinel lymph node excision and interferon therapy (in 2010) was contraindicated because of her cardiac insufficiency. We recommended a careful and intensified follow-up.

Key points
- Nodular melanoma does not show an association to a fair skin type.
- Nodular melanoma has a more aggressive tumor biology compared to superficial spreading melanoma.
- Secondary nodular melanoma is as aggressive as primary nodular melanoma.
- Comorbidities may exclude certain systemic tumor therapies.

References

1. Pizzichetta MA, Massi D, Mandalà M, Queirolo P, Stanganelli I, De Giorgi V, Ghigliotti G, Cavicchini S, Quaglino P, Corradin MT, Rubegni P, Alaibac M, Astorino S, Ayala F, Magi S, Mazzoni L, Manganoni MA, Talamini R, Serraino D, Palmieri G. Italian Melanoma Intergroup (IMI). Clinicopathological predictors of recurrence in nodular and superficial spreading cutaneous melanoma: a multivariate analysis of 214 cases. J Transl Med. 2017;15(1):227.
2. Langholz B, Richardson J, Rappaport E, Waisman J, Cockburn M, Mack T. Skin characteristics and risk of superficial spreading and nodular melanoma (United States). Cancer Causes Control. 2000;11(8):741–50.

Index